Pocket Nurse Guide to
Basic Skills and Procedures

Pocket Nurse Guide to Basic Skills and Procedures

Anne Perry, R.N., M.S.N.

Assistant Professor, School of Nursing
St. Louis University
St. Louis, Missouri

Patricia A. Potter, R.N., M.S.N.

Assistant Director of Nursing Service
Barnes Hospital
St. Louis, Missouri

Illustrated

The C. V. Mosby Company

St. Louis • Toronto • Princeton   1986

MOSBY

A TRADITION OF PUBLISHING EXCELLENCE

Editor: Alison Miller
Developmental editor: Linda L. Duncan
Manuscript editor: George B. Stericker, Jr.
Designer: Diane M. Beasley
Production: Jeanne Genz

Cover and text photography by G. Robert Bishop, 1985

Printed in the United States of America

The C.V. Mosby Company
11830 Westline Industrial Drive, St. Louis, Missouri 63146

ISBN 0-8016-3974-3

C/D/D   9   8   7   6   5   4   3   2

Preface

The *Pocket Nurse Guide to Basic Skills and Procedures* is a quick reference tool for use by both students and practitioners in the clinical setting. It contains 101 skills, many of which nurses will employ on a daily basis in their practice.

Organization

Skills and procedures are grouped according to specialty areas (e.g., medications, fluids, diagnostic procedures). Each skill is presented in an easy-to-read format that includes

1. The purpose for performing each skill
2. A list of actual or potential nursing diagnoses
3. A list of equipment needed
4. A step-by-step outline of the skill with rationales for every step

The skill concludes with helpful information including nurse alerts, client teaching, and pediatric and geriatric considerations.

Special Features

Because an integral part of any nurse's practice is to formulate nursing diagnoses that will in turn help her plan care for her clients, an appendix of approved nursing diagnoses with definitions is provided.

Supplements

Readers are encouraged to refer to Potter-Perry *Fundamentals of Nursing* and Perry-Potter *Clinical Nursing Skills and Techniques* for more in-depth discussion of the material presented here.

Contents

PRELIMINARY
SKILLS

Admission Into the Health Care System

Admission into a health care system can be very stressful. The client meets many staff members throughout the process. His living routines and family relationships have been disrupted by the illness or injury. Diagnostic testing and the numerous admission assessments can be threatening. Often the client feels like a number moving through a maze of health care services.

Upon admission into an agency it is important to familiarize clients with institutional policies and to provide therapeutic support as needed. Inclusion of friends or family into the admission process can be helpful. Once a client reaches a nursing division, it is important for the nurse to collect all the information needed to institute an individualized plan of care.

Potential Nursing Diagnoses

As clients enter the health care system, they will present multiple nursing diagnoses. The influence of the admission process itself may be a contributing factor in the following diagnoses:

> Anxiety related to hospitalization, impending diagnostic and/or treatment procedures, or separation from support persons
>
> Fear related to unknown health status

Equipment

Admission office
Necessary admitting forms

Identification band
General consent form
Nursing unit
Personal care items: bed pan and urinal, wash basin, bath towel and washcloth, toiletry items, tissue paper, water pitcher and glass, emesis basin
Assessment forms
Equipment to perform physical assessment: scale, watch with second hand, thermometer, sphygmomanometer, urine collection cup, additional equipment as needed by type of assessment

Steps	Rationale
Admitting Area	
1. Welcome client and escort him and his family to interviewing area.	Helps relieve anxiety of anticipating first encounter with agency personnel. Interviewing area provides privacy for client.
2. Acquire identifying information, including client's Full legal name Age Birthdate Address Next of kin Physician Religion Previous admissions	Used in all of client's medical records to ensure correct legal identification.
3. Apply identification band to client's wrist containing Client's full legal name Hospital or agency number Physician Birthdate Be sure that band is secure.	Serves as means to officially identify client when therapies or procedures are performed (e.g., medication administration, surgical procedures, x-ray examinations).

Steps	Rationale
4. Instruct client (or legal guardian) to read general consent form for treatment. Assess client's understanding of consent form. ■ Request client (or family member) to sign form if he agrees to be admitted for treatment.	After signing a general consent form, client gives agency right to perform routine procedures and therapies, select room placement, and provide required nursing care.
5. Provide any brochures that describe purpose and organization of agency as well as policies or rules that affect client's conduct.	American Hospital Association's ''Patient's Bill of Rights'' states that client must have access to this information.
6. Assign a room on basis of client's condition, health care needs, and personal preferences.	Clients requiring frequent observation and therapy should be close to central nursing station. Consideration of client's personal preferences during room selection minimizes anxiety and prevents conflict with other clients. Room environment can provide sensory stimulation for sensorially deprived clients.
7. Direct client to area where technicians in admitting office will collect routine blood specimens and perform chest x-ray and electrocardiographic examinations. ■ Instruct client on method for collecting urine specimen.	Routine diagnostic testing serves to screen clients for presence of common physical alterations. Specimen may be collected in admitting area or on nursing division.

Steps	Rationale
8. Notify nursing division of client's admission.	Allows nursing personnel to prepare room and obtain necessary equipment for client's arrival.
■ Report client's name, assigned room and bed, admitting physician, diagnosis, and pertinent information relating to client's condition (e.g., IV line infusing, need for oxygen).	Client may be admitted directly from emergency room.
9. Transport client and family members to nursing division, using an escort.	A member of hospital staff should accompany client to his room to ensure safe arrival.
10. On nursing division, introduce client and his family to nurse who is assuming client's care.	Provides client a sense of personalization during admission process.
11. Share with nursing staff pertinent observations about client's behaviors or level of knowledge regarding need for health care.	Promotes continuity of care so nursing staff can assist client in coping with new environment and procedures of care.

Nursing Division

Steps	Rationale
1. Wash hands.	Prevents spread of microorganisms.
2. Prepare assigned room with necessary equipment and personal care items.	Availability of equipment for personal care promotes client comfort by preventing unnecessary delays during care delivery.
3. Prepare client's bed by adjusting it to lowest horizontal position. Turn down top sheet and spread.	Makes it easier and safer for client to get into bed.

Steps	Rationale
4. Greet client and his family cordially. Introduce yourself by name and job title, telling client you are responsible for his care.	Reduces anxiety client may feel regarding admission. Awareness of which nurse is responsible for his care expedites requests client may have.
5. Escort client and family members to assigned room. Introduce them to roommate if semiprivate room is assigned.	Orientation begins with introduction to roommate.
6. Assess client's general appearance, noting signs or symptoms of physical distress.	If client is experiencing any acute physical problems, routine admission procedures should be postponed until these are cared for.
7. Check physician's orders for any treatment measures that should be initiated immediately.	Delay in initiation of therapies can cause worsening of client's condition.
8. Assess client's and family member's psychological status by noting nonverbal behaviors and verbal responses to greetings and explanations.	Client's level of anxiety influences his ability to adapt to health care environment.
9. Orient client to nursing division: ■ Introduce staff members who enter room. ■ Explain who head nurse or clinical nurse of division is and that person's role in solving problems. ■ Explain visiting hours and their purpose. ■ Discuss smoking policy.	Promotes understanding of agency policies and procedures. Family members' willingness to follow visiting hour policy ensures that client will receive adequate rest.

Steps	Rationale
▪ Demonstrate how to use equipment in room (e.g., bed, over-bed table, lighting).	Client safety depends on understanding of policies and how to use equipment correctly.
▪ Show client how to use nurse call light.	
▪ Escort client to bathroom (if able to ambulate).	
▪ Explain hours for meal time and nourishments.	
▪ Describe services available (e.g., chaplain visitation, gift shop, activity therapy).	
▪ Explain areas where client and family might visit (e.g., cafeteria, lounge, recreation room).	
▪ Warn client against keeping large sums of money or valuables in own room in agency	Because clients are often required to leave their rooms during day, there is risk of money or valuables being stolen.
▪ Inform client about procedure for acquiring television or radio.	
10. Collect any valuables client wishes to have placed in agency safe. Place articles in specially labeled and sealed envelope. Instruct client to sign statement releasing agency of responsibility for valuables.	Only way client can be protected from theft.

Steps	Rationale
11. Explain to client that admitting process will include a nursing history and physical examination. Request client to change into appropriate gown. Provide privacy.	Keeping client informed of procedures and their purpose minimizes anxiety. Hospital gown or pajamas makes it easier to expose body parts during examination.
12. Assist client with hanging or storing clothing in closet or locker.	Basic to most persons' self-image is keeping personal items neat and properly stored.
13. If client prefers, family members may stay in room during history taking; otherwise, escort family to waiting area.	Client may be embarrassed by sharing personal information about his health with family members.
14. Wash hands.	Reduces transmission of microorganisms.
15. Prepare equipment for nursing history and assessment.	Prevents delays that might increase client's anxiety or fatigue.
16. Weigh client and record his height.	Determines baseline values and reveals any recent change in weight.
17. Assist client to assume comfortable position in bed or in bedside chair.	Relieves anxiety and thereby increases accuracy of findings.
18. Assess client's vital signs.	Provides baseline measurement to compare with future findings and discloses any alterations from normal expected range.
19. Obtain nursing history: Client's perceptions of illness Past medical history Presenting signs and symptoms	Provides data necessary to develop individualized plan of care based on client's identified health problems.

Steps	Rationale
Risk factors for illness	
History of allergies	Alerts nurses to substances to
(Nurse provides client an allergy band, similar in size to an identification band, that lists all foods, drugs, or substances to which client is allergic.)	which client is allergic. Prevents accidental administration of substances when client is confused or nonresponsive.
Medication history (If client brings medications to agency, nurse instructs him to take them home; otherwise, medications are stored on division for safekeeping.)	Therapeutic drug administration depends on correct dosages and proper timing as well as avoidance of drug incompatibilities.
Alterations in activities of daily living	Identifying client and family needs early helps in planning
Family resources and support	for eventual discharge from agency.
Potential risk factors for eventual discharge	
20. Conduct physical assessment of appropriate body systems.	Provides objective data for identifying client's health problems.
21. Instruct client on proper technique to provide urine specimen. ■ Label specimen and attach requisition form.	Urinalysis is a basic test to screen for renal and metabolic problems, fluid and electrolyte alterations, and lower urinary tract alterations.
22. Explain to client that technicians will be obtaining blood specimens and performing chest x-ray and electrocardiographic examinations (if not performed in admitting office).	CBC is routine test used to screen for anemias. Blood typing and cross-match are necessary for clients undergoing surgery or who are expected to receive blood transfusions. Chest x-ray screens for preexisting lung disease. Electrocardiogram screens for conduction defects of heart.

Steps	Rationale
23. Inform client about any planned procedures or treatments scheduled for next shift or day (e.g., visit by physician, additional x-rays, dietary restrictions).	Client has right to be informed of any procedures or treatments that he will undergo. Being able to anticipate planned therapies minimizes anxiety.
24. Provide client opportunity to ask questions about any procedure or therapies.	Helps clarify any misconceptions.
25. Allow client and family time together alone.	Admission procedure can be stressful and fatiguing. Client and family often have decisions to make or concerns to share before visitation ends.
26. Be sure call light is within reach, bed is in low position, and side rails are raised.	Provides for client safety.
27. Wash hands.	Reduces transmission of microorganisms.
28. Record history and assessment findings on appropriate forms.	Prompt and thorough documentation prevents deletion of data.
29. Notify physician of client's admission and report any unusual findings.	Client's condition may require immediate medical intervention.
30. Begin to develop nursing care plan.	Provides for continuity of individualized care.

Nurse Alert

When a critically ill client reaches a hospital's nursing division, extensive examination and treatment procedures become necessary almost immediately. Time constraints thus may force the nurse to forego certain steps in the admission process.

Client Teaching

Teaching should center on a discussion of agency procedures and routines as well as activities that the client can expect to experience during the initial days of hospitalization.

Pediatric Considerations

Thorough explanation of the hospital experience and related procedures will reduce a child's fear of the unknown. Ideally children should be prepared for hospitalization before admission, either by parents or by the nursing staff. A tour of hospital facilities and the use of dolls, puppet shows, or specially produced children's films to demonstrate procedures are techniques that will help the child understand hospitalization.

Geriatric Considerations

An elderly person who is to be admitted into a long-term care facility or nursing home often undergoes extensive screening. When such a person enters the hospital, it is very important to orient him to his new surroundings. Gradual loss of sensory perception places the elderly client at risk of sensory overload, resulting in confusion or feelings of isolation.

Discharge From a Health Care Agency

The discharge process involves all members of the health care team. It begins from the time the client enters the health care system. The nursing staff plays an active role in identifying the client's needs throughout his illness so the actual discharge will come as no surprise to anyone. The availability of family members as a resource for care, the extent of a client's physical disability, the predictable need for supplies or equipment at home, and the home environment itself are just some of the factors that nurses will need to assess before the client's discharge. When skilled nursing care is required in the home, nursing staff makes referrals to appropriate health care agencies or works with family members to attain the skills necessary for the client's care. Ongoing communication between all health team members ensures a well-planned discharge process.

Potential Nursing Diagnoses

Ideally clients discharged will have their nursing diagnoses resolved by the time they leave the health care agency. Nursing diagnoses that pose greater risks for the client if discharge planning is not comprehensive include the following:

Self-care deficit related to physical restrictions

Knowledge deficit pertaining to health care practices

Potential for injury related to environmental barriers in the home

Anxiety related to impending discharge

Equipment

Necessary instructional materials
Any ordered prescriptions
Discharge summary form
Utility cart
Wheelchair

Steps	Rationale
Day of Admission	
1. Assess client's health care needs for discharge. Use nursing history, care plan, and ongoing assessments.	The plan for discharge begins at admission and continues throughout course of a client's stay in the agency. It facilitates evental adjustment to home setting.
2. Assess client's and family members' needs for health teaching related to therapies to be administered at home, restrictions resulting from health alterations, complications to be observant for.	Client's and family's understanding of health care needs will improve likelihood of successfully achieving self-care at home. Inclusion of family members in teaching sessions provides client with an available resource when at home.
3. Evaluate with client and family any environmental factors in home setting that might interfere with self-care activities.	Environmental barriers may pose risks to client's safety as result of limitation created by client's illness or need for certain therapies.
4. Assess client's acceptance of health problems and related restrictions.	Client's acceptance of health status can affect his willingness to adhere to therapies and/or restrictions after discharge.
5. Consult with other health team members (e.g., dietitian, social worker) regarding client's needs on discharge.	Members of all health care disciplines should collaborate to determine client's needs and functional abilities.

Steps	Rationale
6. Collaborate with physician in assessing need for referral to skilled home health agencies.	Clients eligible for home health care are confined to home as a result of illness, are under a physician's supervision, or require skilled nursing care on an intermittent basis.
7. Ask client or family members for suggestions on ways to prepare for discharge.	Client should become part of discharge planning team. He may be able to identify additional needs for support or resources that your assessment did not reveal.
8. Suggest methods for altering physical arrangement of home environment to meet client's needs.	Client's level of independence can be maintained within an environment conducive to his safety and ability to retain function. Advanced preparation may be needed before client actually returns home.
9. Offer client and family information about community health care resources.	Community resources often include services that client or family cannot provide.
10. Conduct teaching sessions with client and family as soon as possible during hospitalization on such topics as Signs and symptoms of complications Injections, wound care, transfer techniques, colostomy care Medications, diet, exercise Restrictions imposed by illness or surgery	Gives client and family opportunities to practice new skills, ask questions about therapies, and obtain necessary feedback from you to ensure that learning has occurred.

Steps	Rationale
11. Complete any referral forms indicating client's health care needs as well as existing functional abilities.	Continuity of health care is ensured through communication of individualized plan to all health team members.

Day of Discharge

1. Provide client and family an opportunity to ask questions or discuss issues related to health care needs at home.	Allows for final clarification of information previously discussed. Helps relieve client's anxiety.
2. Check physician's discharge orders for prescriptions, change in treatments, or need for special appliances.	Discharge is authorized only by physician. Early check of orders permits you to attend to any last-minute treatments or procedures in advance of actual discharge.
3. Determine if client or family member has arranged for transport home.	Client's condition at discharge will determine method for transport home.
4. Offer assistance as client dresses into own clothes and packs all personal belongings. Provide privacy as needed.	Promotes client comfort.
5. Make a final check of closets and drawers to be sure that all of client's belongings have been removed.	Prevents loss of client's personal items.
6. Obtain copy of valuables list signed by client at admission and have security personnel or appropriate administrator deliver valuables to client. Have client put initials on receipt.	Client's signature on list will verify receipt of items.

Steps	Rationale
7. Be sure that all valuables are accounted for.	Relieves agency of liability for any losses.
8. Check that client has any prescriptions or medications ordered by physician. Review with him and a family member drug dosage and precautions as well as other pertinent information.	Review of drug information provides feedback to determine client's success in learning about medications.
9. Contact agency's business office to determine if client needs to finalize arrangements for payment of bill. Arrange for client or family member to visit office.	A source of concern for many clients is whether agency has accepted insurance or other payment forms.
10. Acquire utility cart to move client's belongings. Obtain wheelchair for clients unable to ambulate. Clients leaving by ambulance will be transported on ambulance stretchers.	Provides for safe transport.
11. Use proper body mechanics and transfer techniques in assisting client to wheelchair or stretcher.	Prevents injury to you and to client.
12. Escort client to entrance of agency where source of transportation is waiting.	Agency policy requires escort to ensure client's safe exit.
13. Lock wheelchair wheels. Assist client in tranferring to automobile or transport vehicle. Help family member place personal belongings inside vehicle.	Agency's liability ends once client is safely in vehicle.

Steps	Rationale
14. Return to division and notify admitting or appropriate department of time client was discharged.	Allows agency to prepare for admission of next client.
15. Complete discharge summary in clients' medical record.	Essential for documenting client's status at time of departure from agency.

Nurse Alert

Do not ignore clients who fail to pose an obvious need for discharge planning. Too often clients with short stays in a health care agency may not receive teaching or necessary referrals until the day of discharge.

Client Teaching

Individualize any discussions or demonstrations so the client can easily apply what he learns to the home setting.

Pediatric Considerations

A child's developmental age must be considered before attempting to prepare him for any home-care skills. Parents are most commonly involved in any preparation for the child's discharge.

Geriatric Considerations

Elderly clients with mobility restrictions or sensory limitations will benefit from the installation of safety and/or assistive devices (such as grab bars around toilets, new lighting in bathrooms, or chair height adjustments to make bending easier).

Writing a Nursing Diagnosis

A nursing diagnosis is a statement of the client's potential or actual health problem that the nurse is licensed and competent to treat. The overall purpose of the nursing diagnosis is to interpret assessment data and thus identify health problems involving the client, the family, and significant others.

The diagnostic process includes three major elements: analysis and interpretation of data, identification of client problems, and formulation of nursing diagnoses.

1. Analysis and interpretation of data require data validation and data clustering. Validation involves determining the relationship between assessment data and health needs and determining their accuracy. Data clustering is the process that the nurse uses to group related data.
2. Identification of client problems involves determining what the general health problems are and whether they are actual or potential problems. When identifying client needs the nurse must consider all aspects of the nursing assessment.
3. Formulation of actual nursing diagnoses identifies the specific nursing care need of each client. Individualization of such needs allows the nurse to develop a specific nursing care plan for each of her clients.

Clients entering a health care agency may have more than one nursing diagnosis based on their individual health care problem. The Appendix, at the end of this text, includes the nursing diagnoses currently accepted by the North American Nursing Diagnosis Association (NANDA).

Steps	Rationale
1. Validate pertinent data identified during history taking and physical assessment. Validation can be achieved from secondary source of information such as client, reexamination, or results of laboratory tests.	Determines whether data gathered during assessment are complete and accurate.

EXAMPLE
Client states he gets short of breath climbing stairs. *Data validation:* Client is requested to climb stairs in his home. After climbing six stairs, he shows respiratory rate increase from 18 to 32 breaths/min. Nasal flaring and diaphoresis are present, pulse rate is increased from 82 to 116, BP is stable.

Steps	Rationale
2. Group related data, which are generally signs and symptoms indicating general health problem. Related data are clustered as regards client's mental or emotional status, individual body systems, risk factors, family data, and community factors.	Clustering of data encourages you to identify patterns for health care. In addition, clustering identifies related changes in client's needs and ultimately leads to formulation of nursing diagnoses.

EXAMPLE
Client states that he has shortness of breath with exertion. *Data clustering:* Respiratory rate is increased from 18 to 32 breaths/min. Pulse rate is

Steps	Rationale

increased from 82 to 116 with exertion. Nasal flaring and diaphoresis are present with exertion.

3. List general health care problems of client.
   a. Actual health care problem: one that is currently perceived by client
   b. Potential health care problem: one that client is at risk of developing

Allows beginning nurse to identify broad general nursing problems.

EXAMPLE
- *Actual* health care problem—shortness of breath with exertion
- *Potential* health care problem—reduced activity level

4. Write nursing diagnosis in two parts.
   a. Problem: actual or potential client need that can be resolved by nursing interventions

   Lists general nursing diagnostic (NANDA) label.

   b. Cause: direct or contributing factor in development of client need

   Helps to individualize nursing diagnosis and subsequent plan of care.

EXAMPLE
- *Problem*—ineffective breathing pattern related to *cause* (exertion)
- *Problem*—potential activity intolerance related to *cause* (shortness of breath)

Steps	Rationale
5. Reevaluate list of individualized nursing diagnoses developed for each client contact.	As client's needs change, nursing diagnoses are modified. Some may no longer be relevant, while new ones may need to be developed.

Writing a Nursing Care Plan

The nursing care plan is a written guideline for client care so the specifics of nursing care can be quickly communicated to all nursing personnel. Written nursing care plans document the individual health care needs of the client as determined by assessment and the nursing diagnoses. During planning, priorities and goals are formulated to coordinate nursing care, promote continuity of care, and list outcome criteria that will be used in the evaluation of nursing care. In addition, the written care plan communicates to other nurses and health professionals specific individualized nursing therapies.

Steps	Rationale
1. Determine goals of nursing care for each nursing diagnosis.	Nursing goal is specific aim planned by you to assist client in achieving maximum level of wellness. Setting goals is an activity that includes family and significant others, as well as the client. Ultimately it determines the outcome of the nursing intervention.

EXAMPLE

Nursing Diagnoses	*Goals*
Potential ineffective coping related to fear of medical diagnosis	Mr. Brown to ask pertinent questions about cancer
Potential ineffective airway clearance postoperatively related to abdominal incision	Mr. Brown's lungs to remain clear postoperatively

Steps	Rationale
2. Establish priorities of care. Rank nursing diagnoses and goals in order of importance. Priorities are classified as high, intermediate, or low.	High-priority nursing diagnoses reflect emergency or immediate needs of client. High priorities occur in psychological as well as physiological dimensions. Intermediate-priority nursing diagnoses reflect nonemergency non–life-threatening needs of client. Low-priority nursing diagnoses reflect client goals not directly related to his specific illness or prognosis.

EXAMPLE
Nursing Diagnoses

Rationale for Priority Setting

High Priority
Potential ineffective coping related to fear of medical diagnosis of cancer
Potential ineffective airway clearance postoperatively related to abdominal incision

Dealing with this early will help Mr. Brown prepare for surgery and his postoperative restorative care.
Because of this, you will institute preventive client education preoperatively.

Intermediate Priority
Alteration in bowel elimination related to diarrhea of unknown cause

Does not affect client's immediate physiological or emotional status. Also, future surgery will assist you in resolving diagnosis.

Low Priority
Potential for chronic respiratory tract infection related to history of smoking for 20 years

Reflects long-term needs of client.

Steps	Rationale
3. For each nursing diagnosis, write projected outcomes anticipated from nursing action. Projected outcomes should reflect goals established in Step 1.	Change in client's condition that care plan is designed to bring about. Includes degree of wellness and need for continuing care, medications, support, counseling, and education.

EXAMPLE

Nursing Diagnosis	*Projected Outcome*
Potential ineffective airway clearance postoperatively related to abdominal incision	Lungs clear to auscultation

Goal
Mr. Brown's lungs to remain clear postoperatively

Steps	Rationale
4. Write specific implementation measures. Should include when, how much, where, etc.	Must be specific so there is continuity of care from one nurse to another.
5. Modify nursing care plan based on nursing assessment as client's status or needs change.	Continually individualizes nursing care for client based on his changing needs.

Communicating During the Orientation Phase

Communication is the means to understanding and caring for the client. Without effective communication skills the nurse is often ineffective with the care she provides. For example, a nurse cannot administer an injection as effectively unless she knows how to recognize the client's apprehension and how to explain the procedure in a way that calms the client. Communication skills are a vital part of every interaction that goes on between nurse and client. When effective communication is practiced and integrated into the nurse's care, it becomes a powerful tool in all aspects of nursing.

This skill can be useful to the nurse in the process of planned purposeful communication with a client. It reviews the basic steps used during the orientation phase of the nurse-client relationship. It is important to remember that a nurse's interaction may be brief or long and may require different techniques depending on the purpose or situations involved in the interaction. Any communication with a client must be through a relationship based on mutual trust so a meaningful interaction occurs.

Potential Nursing Diagnoses

Skills of effective communication are necessary for nurses in dealing with clients who may have virtually any nursing diagnosis. However, certain diagnoses call for greater communication skills than others. Examples of these include the following:

   Anxiety related to hospitalization, impending surgery, separation from family

Fear related to impending surgery or therapy

Knowledge deficit related to no previous experience with illness

Impaired verbal communication related to sensory deficit or different cultural language

Impaired verbal communication related to surgical procedures: laryngectomy

Steps	Rationale
1. Determine type and availability of environment most conducive to interaction:	Certain environments are more conducive to therapeutic interactions than others.
▪ Choose private environment for certain tasks and interactions (e.g., discussion of planned therapy, fear of death, concerns over family members).	Privacy is less threatening to client. Promotes freer expression of feelings.
2. Reduce or eliminate sources of distraction or interuptions in environment.	Ongoing activity, loud noises, and interruptions may hinder message that was intended.
3. Take care of client's physical discomfort or needs before beginning discussion (e.g., positioning, liquids or food, pain relief, assistance to bathroom).	Will decrease client's distraction.
4. Create initial climate of warmth and acceptance:	Facilitates more open exchange.
▪ Decrease your own anxiety by preparing for interaction, pausing and collecting thoughts before entering room, relaxing by taking several deep breaths.	Helps decrease client's anxiety by seeing you in calm relaxed state.

Steps	Rationale
5. Sit in comfortable chair near client. Make sure that you are at same eye level, facing each other and maintaining good eye contact.	Physical attending provides nonverbal message to client that you are interested in him.
■ Maintain "open" position (avoid crossing your legs and arms), leaning toward client and remaining relatively relaxed.	Demonstrates willingness to communicate.
6. Listen to or observe client's nonverbal behavior. (This often carries emotional dimension of messages.) Listen to client's verbal behavior. Take time to listen. Teach yourself to concentrate. Don't interrupt. Listen "between the lines."	Psychological attending makes you more alert to client's true message. It is also congruent with your nonverbal message conveyed in physical attending.
7. Introduce yourself and provide information.	Assists in orientation.
■ Tell him of hospital or agency facilities and environment (e.g., call light, bed adjustments, cabinet space, special equipment).	Increases client's capability of managing environment.
■ Give him any informational pamphlets (e.g., orientation to area of care, services available, treatment and/or testing procedures).	Reinforces teaching and allows client to review material.
■ Advise him on beginning plan of care (e.g., procedures that need to be completed, activities, gathering specimens).	Increases client's participation in care because of better understanding.

Steps	Rationale

■ Provide general schedule for day.

Helps both you and client plan day or alter schedule.

8. Help client manage anxiety by providing information regarding what he can expect, checking on and acknowledging him frequently, encouraging him to participate in usual activities as much as possible, assisting him in expressing concerns and fears.

In orientation phase anxiety may be related to fear of unknown or changes and interruptions in usual activities or life-style.

9. Use communication techniques and tools that facilitate orientation phase (Egan, 1975):

Assists in establishing rapport with client that promotes free exchange of information.

■ *Accurate empathy.* Listen to message. Respond frequently but briefly to message; respond to both feelings and content. Attend carefully to signs that either confirm or deny accuracy of your response.

Communicates understanding of client's feelings and experiences. Client senses your interest in what he has to say.

■ *Respect.* Be "for" the client. Be willing and available to work with him. Recognize his uniqueness. Practice psychological and physical attending. Suspend critical judgments. Express warmth. Give recognition by greeting client or indicate awareness of change or efforts being made by client.

Communicates positive regard for client.

Steps	Rationale
• *Genuineness*. Be non-defensive. Be consistent in what you think, feel, and say. Be spontaneous but not impulsive. Avoid facade.	You must be basically yourself and allow client to be himself.
• *Concreteness*. Do not let client ramble. Ask for more specific information. Avoid vagueness ("I noticed that you have been staying in your bed today"). Begin to explore ("Tell me more about . . . ."). Clarification ("I'm not sure I follow."). Paraphrase or restate client's message.	By speaking about specific experiences, specific behaviors, and/or specific feelings, client is likely to speak of specific problems with specific solutions.
10. Use questions carefully: • Use open-ended and nonthreatening questions as much as possible.	Client is usually more willing to express himself.
• Avoid numerous direct questions; avoid using why and how as much as possible.	Numerous direct questions and why and how questions can be intimidating and annoying to client.
11. Avoid communication breakdown in orientation phase, caused by: Rushing into working phase before establishment of initial trust and rapport.	This occurs when message is not received, or is distorted, or is not understood. Client may not be ready and may resist working with you.
Uncomfortable silence. Your anxiety increasing with client's anxiety. Vagueness in answering client's questions.	Increases client's anxiety. May hinder development of trust and confidence. Client may begin to lack confidence in your ability.

Steps	Rationale
12. Summarize with client what has been discussed during interaction:	Signals close of interaction, allows you and client to depart with same idea, and provides sense of closure at completion of discussion.
"Let me see if I have everything we talked about. We reviewed your treatment plan and what you will need to do. You expressed concern about your length of stay at the hospital and not being able to return to work immediately. Is there anything else?"	
13. Record in nurse's notes communication pertinent to client's health, responses to illness or therapies, and acceptance of health care measures.	Provides data for assessment of client's needs and problems.
▪ Include behaviors or nonverbal cues that reflect client's refusal or acceptance of health care measures and response toward therapies.	Documents client's response to nursing care.

Nurse Alert

Throughout any discussion with a client it is important for the nurse to observe his nonverbal behavioral responses. Nonverbal feedback reveals the client's willingness to communicate and can help the nurse redirect communication when the interaction is faltering.

Client Teaching

Effective communication is essential for any form of client education. While the nurse attempts to establish a relationship with a client, she can also determine his readiness and ability to learn.

Pediatric Considerations

A nurse must be able to communicate effectively not only with a child but with the child's parents as well. Nonverbal communication tends to convey the most significant messages to children. Children are very alert to a nurse's feelings, attitudes, and anxiety. The nurse must establish a sense of trust with the child. A quiet, unhurried, and confident voice works best with children of any age.

Geriatric Considerations

When communicating with elderly clients, remember that they bring a world of experiences with them. Aging does not automatically impair intelligence or insight. The nurse will have to adjust communication techniques for those clients with sensory or perceptual alterations (for example, reduced hearing or vision, poor attention span, impaired memory).

Communicating With the Anxious Client

It is quite common for a nurse to encounter a client who is experiencing anxiety. A newly diagnosed illness, separation from family, the discomfort of diagnostic and/or treatment procedures, the threat of surgery, and the expectations of life changes are examples of factors that can cause a client to become anxious. How effectively the nurse can communicate with a client will affect the extent to which his anxiety can be relieved. The communication methods in this skill can assist the nurse in helping an anxious client clarify the factors causing anxiety and cope with anxiety-producing situations more effectively.

Potential Nursing Diagnoses

The verbal and nonverbal cues that can direct a nurse's recognition to the client's anxiety may result in any of the following nursing diagnoses:

Anxiety related to alterations in life-style

Impaired verbal communication related to anxiety

Ineffective individual coping related to impending surgery or diagnostic findings

Steps	Rationale
1. Provide quiet calm environment, away from groups of people and activity.	Decreasing stimuli can have a calming result.
2. Allow ample personal space.	There is direct correlation between amount of personal space needed and level of anxiety. Nature of nurse-client relationship may determine personal space needed.
3. Acknowledge and take care of anxious client's physical and emotional discomfort but avoid dwelling on physical complaints.	Anxiety can be very unpleasant emotional experience and sometimes is expressed in physical discomfort or complaints.
4. Create climate of warmth and acceptance: ■ Maintain composure during interaction.	Can have calming effect on client.
■ Stay with client or check frequently if he is experiencing extreme anxiety.	Provides reassurance to anxious client.
■ Demonstrate genuineness and respect.	Allows client to be himself and creates attitude that communicates positive regard between you and client.
5. Use physical attending:	Nonverbal message to client conveys your interest.
■ Sit in comfortable chair near client. ■ Maintain same eye level with client, facing him. Maintain "open" position (avoid crossing your legs and arms), leaning toward client and remaining relaxed.	

Steps	Rationale
6. Use psychological attending: ■ Listen to client's verbal behavior. Take time to listen; concentrate. Don't interrupt; listen "between the lines"	Enables you to be more alert to client's message.
7. Provide brief simple introduction: introduce yourself and state who you are. Explain purpose of interaction.	Anxiety may limit amount of information client can understand.
8. Use communication techniques and tools to respond to an anxious client: ■ Anticipate needs.	Client may ignore his needs. Meeting needs makes him more comfortable.
■ Make replies simple, clear, and related to situation.	Client's perception and attention may be limited.
■ Avoid introducing anything new.	Client may become overwhelmed by new situation or experience.
■ Limit amount of decision making.	Prevents further escalation of anxiety.
■ Provide for physical activity, such as walking.	Requires little concentration and can help decrease anxiety.
■ Use accurate empathy. State what you understand message to be (e.g., "I understand you to say . . ."; "I hear you saying . . ."; "I sense that . . . ").	Communicating understanding often has a de-escalating effect on anxiety.
■ Use concreteness.	Can often eliminate vagueness associated with anxiety.

Steps	Rationale
9. Use questions and responses based on hierarchy: description of experience, thoughts about experience, feelings that experience generates:	Aids client in describing event and clarifying his thoughts and feelings.

Nurse: What happened? I sense that you are upset about something.

Client: The doctor was just here. (Describes experience)

Nurse: Tell me more about what happened. (Offers to explore experience further)

Client: He said I won't be getting to go home tomorrow and that I will have to stay until I am able to eat more.

Nurse: What do you think about that? (Requests thoughts about experience)

Client: Well, I know he is right. I haven't been eating, but I was counting on going home.

Nurse: What are your feelings? (Offers to explore the experience further)

Client: I'm disappointed and angry, but I need to stay here for now.

Steps	Rationale
10. Don't let communication breakdown occur with anxious client: belittling thoughts and feelings associated with anxiety (e.g., "There is no reason why you should feel this way"); ignoring his discomfort connected with anxiety; ignoring him; getting angry with him (e.g., "You have to stop this right now!"); being unable to acknowledge and control your own anxiety.	Communication breakdown can increase anxiety and feelings of isolation.
11. Record in nurse's notes cause of client's anxiety and any exhibited signs and symptoms or behaviors:	Documents nature of client's problem and his response.
▪ Include methods used to relieve anxiety and client's response.	Provides guidelines for other nurses to continue interaction.

Nurse Alert

The nurse's interaction can increase a client's anxiety if techniques are not used appropriately. Be alert for signs of anxiety. Physical signs can include dry mouth, sweaty palms, diarrhea, urinary frequency, increases in the respiratory and heart rate and in blood pressure, headache, nausea, and upset stomach. Behavioral signs of anxiety can include tense voice, difficulty in concentrating, insomnia, loss of appetite, pacing, inability to sit still, wringing of hands, expanding one aspect of the total situation out of proportion, and irritability.

Client Teaching

Teaching should not be conducted when a client is anxious. He will then likely be unable to attend to your instructions.

Pediatric Considerations

Communicate at the child's level by sitting on a low chair, kneeling, squatting, or even sitting on the floor. Preserve physical closeness with the parent if possible by allowing the child to sit on the parent's lap. Use of dolls or toys may help quiet an anxious child. Never perform any procedure on a young child without explaining it clearly in simple language. Use as few words as possible. Be positive and honest with the child. Do not provide too advanced a warning; otherwise, the child's fantasies may heighten his anxiety. Perform the procedure quickly after the explanation.

Geriatric Considerations

Elderly persons can experience considerable stress, but they do not react in the same way as younger persons. Severe anxiety is rare among the elderly. They do not seem to have the energy to fight or flee when stress occurs. Instead, they tend to accept, contemplate, and even show apathy as a means of coping.

Communicating With the Angry Client

In a health care setting a client may be angry over experiences with illness or over problems that existed before he sought health care. It is important for the nurse to understand that in many cases the client's ability to express anger is an essential part of his recovery. For example, the client grieving over loss of a body part must be able to express anger in order to cope effectively.

Anger can represent rejection or disapproval of the nurse's care. The nurse should encourage the client to express anger openly and should not feel threatened by the client's words. When a client becomes angry, the nurse must not allow the emotion to compromise her care of him.

Potential Nursing Diagnoses

The verbal and nonverbal cues that direct a nurse to recognize a client's anger may result in the following nursing diagnoses:

Impaired verbal communication related to feelings of anger

Ineffective individual coping related to anger

Dysfunctional grieving related to physical loss or chronic illness

Steps	Rationale
1. Physically prepare angry client and environment:	
▪ Encourage other people, particularly those who provoke his anger, to leave room or area.	You want client to express his anger, but you do not want to provoke it.
▪ Maintain adequate distance.	Avoids pressuring client. Also you should maintain a safe distance if anger becomes out of control.
▪ Maintain an open exit.	Prevents feeling of being trapped.
▪ Make sure that your gestures are slow and deliberate rather than sudden and abrupt.	Less chance of misinterpretation of message and is less threatening.
▪ Reduce disturbing factors in his room (e.g., noise, drafts, inadequate lighting).	Reduces irritating factors.
▪ Take care of physical and emotional needs and discomforts.	Physical and emotional needs may be factors in client's anger. Sometimes he may not be aware of these needs.
2. Use physical attending:	
▪ Begin with minimal intensity and very gradually increase.	Adequate personal space is very important with an angry client.
▪ Begin with same type of position as client (when possible). Example: If client is standing, you stand. If client is sitting, you sit.	Conveys physically being "in tune" with another.
▪ Gradually move to more relaxed position for both you and client. Example: If standing, eventually sit.	Facilitates less tense or less anxious exchange.

Steps	Rationale
▪ Keep your shoulders slightly down or relaxed.	Uses body language that is less intimidating or threatening.
▪ Look toward client but avoid glaring or eye contact that is too intense.	Less intimidating.
▪ Maintain "open" position. Avoid crossing your legs and arms. Keep hands unclenched and relaxed. Face slightly toward client.	Provides nonverbal cues of acceptance and listening that are congruent with attitude of acceptance.
3. Use psychological attending:	
▪ Avoid defensive listening with an angry client.	In listening defensively instead of normally, you concentrate on your need to defend yourself or reasons why client should not feel angry.
4. Introduce yourself and state who you are. Be brief and to the point.	Often client may not be able to listen or hear details of conversation. He may be concentrating only on his own point of view.
5. Respond to angry client:	
▪ Use therapeutic silence.	Often de-escalates anger, because anger expands emotional and physical energy and client runs out of momentum and energy to maintain anger at high level.
▪ Use responses based on this hierarchy: description of experience, thoughts about experience, feelings that experience has generated.	Assists client in describing event causing anger and clarifying his thoughts and feelings.

Steps	Rationale
▪ Make vague statements more explicit or specific. Client: Nobody cares around here. Nurse: I'm not sure what you mean, Mr. Jones. Could you tell me more? Client: Everybody is just too busy. Nurse: What do you mean, everybody is just too busy? Client: I haven't seen anybody for 3 hours and I need my dressing changed before I go to physical therapy.	Angry client may have difficulty in being specific and needs assistance to do so. To change factors contributing to client's anger, you will often need specific information.
▪ Practice accurate empathy.	This is ability to comprehend and communicate with accuracy thoughts, feelings, and experience of client in such a way that he would say, "Yes, that is exactly where I'm coming from." It is strong anger antidote.
▪ Explore alternatives to situation or feelings of anger.	May alter factors contributing to anger.
▪ Present your perspective or point of view calmly and firmly.	May assist client to understand whole situation or another point of view. Also may assist in getting client to comply or follow through with care.
▪ Use repeated assertion. Firmly repeat original response rather than argue each point.	Can be effective when client ignores, overreacts, or discounts your thoughts or feelings.

Steps	Rationale
6. Use questions carefully:	
■ Make them open-ended and nonthreatening as much as possible.	Client becomes more willing to express himself.
■ Avoid numerous direct questions. Avoid using why and how.	Can intimidate and annoy client.
7. Don't let communication breakdown occur:	
■ Avoid attempts to show client why he should not be angry.	Client will react more to emotions than to reasoning.
■ Avoid aggressiveness or oversubmissive behavior.	Both tend to escalate client's anger.
■ Do not ignore client's anger.	You may lose opportunity to assist client in resolving anger.
■ Avoid trying to "out-talk" or give numerous explanations.	Annoys and irritates client.
8. Record in nurse's notes observations related to anger. Quote client exactly.	Aids in assessing source of client's anger.
■ Include nursing interventions in response to client's anger.	Documents your actions.

Nurse Alert

The nurse's failure to use proper techniques may increase a client's anger. It is important to remove factors contributing to anger (for example, do not ask a visitor to leave the room if the client desires company, cease any attempts to convince the client that he is wrong). Unless a potentially out-of-control situation is defused, the client may hurt himself or someone else.

Client Teaching

Teaching will be ineffective during a period when the client is angry, unless lack of knowledge is the source of his anger. Even then the nurse should limit explanations to simple discussions.

Pediatric Considerations

Anger is commonly expressed more frequently in individuals who are emotionally immature or impulsive (as in children).

Geriatric Considerations

The elderly client who suffers from an organic brain syndrome will often be impulsive and may become frustrated easily. Thus he also can become angry easily.

VITAL SIGNS

Measuring Oral
Temperature

Normally a person's body temperature fluctuates within a relatively narrow range. Under control of the hypothalamus the body's core temperature stays within 0.6° of 37° C (1° of 98.6° F). Alterations may result from disease, infection, prolonged exposure to heat or cold, exercise, and hormonal disturbances. The body adapts to temperature changes by conserving or losing heat depending on the nature of the temperature alteration.

The oral method is the easiest way to obtain an accurate temperature reading. The nurse should delay measurement for 30 minutes if the client has ingested hot or cold liquids or food or has smoked. Each of these can cause false changes in temperature levels. During assessment of body temperature the nurse should consider the client's risks of temperature alterations. Conditions or therapies that can cause temperature alterations include expected or diagnosed infections, open wounds or burns, abnormal white cell count, use of immunosuppressive drugs, injury to the hypothalamus, lengthy exposure to temperature extremes, and reaction to blood products.

Potential Nursing Diagnoses

After assessing the client's temperature and observing for signs and symptoms of temperature alterations, the nurse may make the following nursing diagnoses:

Potential for injury related to infection or drug reaction

Fluid volume deficit related to diaphoresis

Equipment

Oral or stubby mercury-in-glass thermometer
Tissue paper

Steps	Rationale
1. Wash hands.	Reduces transmission of microorganisms.
2. Hold tip of thermometer in your fingertips.	Prevents contamination of bulb to be inserted into client's mouth.
3. If thermometer is stored in a disinfectant solution, rinse it in cold water before using.	Removes potentially irritating disinfectant. Hot water might cause mercury to expand and break bulb.
4. Take soft tissue and wipe thermometer from bulb end toward fingers in a rotating manner. Dispose of tissue.	Rotating friction helps remove microorganisms. Wiping toward fingers prevents contamination of bulb end.
5. Read mercury level, holding thermometer at eye level. (Fig. 1)	Mercury is to be below 35.5° C (96° F). Thermometer reading must be below client's actual temperature before use.

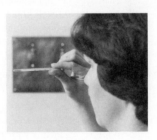

Fig. 1

6. If mercury is above desired level, shake thermometer down. Grasp tip of thermometer securely	Brisk shaking lowers mercury level in glass tube. Standing in open spot prevents breakage of thermometer.

Steps	Rationale
and stand away from any solid objects. Sharply flick wrist downward as though cracking a whip. Continue until reading is at appropriate level.	
7. Ask client to open his mouth and gently place thermometer in sublingual pocket (under tongue) lateral to center of lower jaw.	Heat from superficial blood vessels under the tongue produces temperature reading.
8. Ask client to hold thermometer with lips closed.	Lips hold thermometer in proper position during recording.
9. Leave thermometer in place 3-8 minutes according to agency policy.	Studies disagree as to proper length of time for recording. Nichols and Kucha (1972) recommend 8 minutes for oral glass thermometers. Graves and Markarian (1980) found that glass thermometers kept in place for 8 minutes recorded values on average only 0.07° F higher than those kept in for 3 minutes. Therefore they recommend 3 minutes as more practical.
10. Carefully remove thermometer and read temperature level.	Gentle handling prevents client discomfort.
11. Wipe off any secretions with a soft tissue. Wipe in rotating fashion from tip to bulb. Dispose of tissue.	Prevents contact of microorganisms with your hands. Tip is area of least contamination, bulb area of greatest contamination.
12. Wash thermometer in lukewarm soapy water. Rinse in cool water and dry.	Mechanically removes organic material that can hinder action of disinfectant.

Steps	Rationale
13. Store thermometer in its container after shaking it down again.	Prevents breakage.
14. Record client's temperature in proper chart or flow sheet.	Should be done immediately before it is forgotten.

Nurse Alert

Oral temperature measurement is contraindicated when the thermometer can injure the client or if the client is unable to hold the thermometer properly. Examples of contraindications include infants and small children, clients undergoing oral surgery or with pain in or trauma to the mouth, confused or unconscious clients, mouth breathers, clients with a history of convulsions, and clients with a shaking chill.

Client Teaching

Clients susceptible to temperature alterations should know how to measure their temperatures correctly so they can seek medical attention early when alterations occur. Parents of young children should learn to measure body temperature since children can develop seriously high fevers quickly.

Pediatric Considerations

Oral temperature measurement is not used in infants or small children. Most institutions recommend an age for permitting oral temperatures (for example, after 5 or 6 years). The immaturity of a child's temperature regulation mechanisms can cause sudden changes in body temperature. A newborn's body temperature normally ranges from 35.5° to 37.5° C (96 to 99.5° F).

Geriatric Considerations

Disturbances in temperature regulation that normally occur with aging can cause the elderly client to have a lower than normal body temperature.

Measuring Rectal
Temperature

The nurse measures a client's body temperature rectally when use of an oral thermometer is contraindicated. The rectal site provides a reliable measure of body temperature. However, a client can easily become embarrassed when rectal temperature must be measured. Thus the nurse should take care to consider the client's privacy and comfort.

Certain conditions contraindicate rectal temperature measurement: a newborn infant, a client with rectal surgery or disorder, a client in pelvic or lower extremity traction or cast. Rectal temperature measurement is most reliable in young children.

Potential Nursing Diagnoses

After assessing the client's temperature and observing for signs and symptoms of temperature alterations, the nurse may make the following nursing diagnoses:

Potential for injury related to infection, heat exposure
Fluid volume deficit related to diaphoresis

Equipment

Rectal thermometer
Lubricant
Tissue paper

Steps	Rationale
1. Wash hands.	Reduces transmission of microorganisms.
2. Hold tip of thermometer in your fingertips.	This prevents contamination of the bulb to be inserted into client's rectum.
3. If thermometer is stored in a disinfectant solution, rinse it in cold water before using.	Removes potentially irritating disinfectant. Hot water might cause mercury to expand and break bulb.
4. Wipe thermometer from bulb end toward fingers in a rotating manner. Dispose of tissue.	Rotating friction helps remove microorganisms. Wiping toward fingers prevents contamination of bulb end.
5. Read mercury level.	Mercury should be below 35.5° C (96° F) and below client's actual temperature before use.
6. If mercury is above desired level, shake thermometer down. Grasp upper end of thermometer securely and stand away from any solid objects. Sharply flick wrist downward as though cracking a whip. Continue until reading is at appropriate level.	Brisk shaking lowers mercury level in glass tube. Standing in an open spot away from objects prevents breakage of thermometer.
7. Draw curtains around client's bed or close room door. Keep client's upper body and lower extremities covered.	Maintains client privacy and minimizes embarrassment.
8. Ask adult client to roll over onto his side, assuming Sims' position, with upper leg flexed. Move aside bed linen to expose only anal area. Child may lie prone.	Provides optimal exposure of anal area for correct thermometer placement.

Steps	Rationale
9. Squeeze liberal amount of water-soluble lubricant onto a tissue. Dip thermometer bulb end into lubricant, covering 2.5-3.5 cm (1-1½ inches) for adult or 1.2-2.5 cm (½-1 inch) for infant or child.	Inserting thermometer into lubricant container would contaminate all unused lubricant. Lubrication minimizes trauma to rectal mucosa during insertion.
10. Put disposable glove on your dominant hand.	This step is optional. It helps reduce contact with microorganisms.
11. With your nondominant hand raise client's upper buttock to expose anus. While infant lies prone on a bed or on your lap, gently retract both buttocks with your fingers.	Retracting buttocks fully exposes anus.
12. Gently insert thermometer into anus in direction of umbilicus. Insert 1.2 cm (½ inch) for infant and 3.5 cm (1½ inches) for adult.	Proper insertion ensures adequate exposure to blood vessels in rectal wall.
13. Do not force thermometer. Ask client to take deep breath and blow out. Insert thermometer as client breathes deeply. If you feel resistance, withdraw thermometer immediately.	Gentle insertion prevents trauma to mucosa or breakage of thermometer. Taking deep breath helps to relax anal sphincter.
14. Hold thermometer in place 2-4 minutes according to agency policy. You may have to hold an infant's legs.	Holding thermometer prevents injury to client.
15. Carefully remove thermometer.	Prevents injury to mucosa.

Steps	Rationale
16. Wipe any secretions off with a tissue. Wipe down in a rotating fashion from tip to bulb. Dispose of tissue.	Prevents your contacting microorganisms. Tip is area of least contamination, bulb area of greatest contamination.
17. Wipe client's anal area to remove lubricant or feces.	Provides for client's comfort.
18. Read thermometer.	
19. Help client return to a more comfortable position.	Restores client's comfort.
20. Wash thermometer in lukewarm soapy water and rinse in cool water.	Washing mechanically removes organic material that otherwise might be source of infection.
21. Dry thermometer and return it to its container after shaking it down.	Proper storage prevents breakage.
22. Remove glove by pulling it off at wrist, turning it inside out. Discard glove in proper receptacle.	Avoidance of contact with glove's outer surface minimizes spread of microorganisms
23. Wash your hands.	Reduces transmission of microorganisms.
24. Record client's temperature in proper chart or flow sheet. Signify rectal reading by capital *R*.	Vital signs should be recorded immediately after measurement. *R* prevents later confusion with oral or axillary measurements.

Nurse Alert

Always hold a rectal thermometer while it is in place. Sudden movement by the client could cause the thermometer to break in the rectum.

Client Teaching

Instruct mothers of young children how to position and restrain the child properly during thermometer insertion.

Pediatric Considerations

Rectal temperature recording is contraindicated in newborns. Do not allow infants or young children to kick their legs or roll to the side while the thermometer is in place. The immaturity of a child's temperature regulation mechanisms can cause sudden changes in body temperature. A newborn's body temperature normally ranges between 35.5° and 37.5°C (96° and 99.5° F).

Geriatric Considerations

Disturbances in temperature regulation that normally occur with aging can cause elderly clients to have a lower than normal body temperature. An elderly person may have difficulty flexing his knee or hip to assume the Sims position. In that case, allow him to lie on his side with legs straight.

Measuring Axillary Temperature

The axillary temperature measurement is the safest method for assessing body temperature in a newborn. However, an axillary temperature is the least accurate of the three temperature measurement techniques because the thermometer must be placed against an external body site instead of an internal site. Whenever an oral or rectal thermometer can be safely used, the nurse should avoid using the axillary thermometer.

Potential Nursing Diagnoses

After assessing the client's temperature and observing for signs and symptoms of temperature alterations, the nurse may make the following nursing diagnoses:

Potential for injury related to infection

Fluid volume deficit related to diaphoresis

Equipment

Oral or stubby mercury-in-glass thermometer
Tissue paper

Steps	Rationale
1. Wash hands.	Reduces transmission of microorganisms.
2. Hold upper end of thermometer in your fingertips.	Prevents contamination of the bulb.

Steps	Rationale
3. If thermometer is stored in disinfectant solution, rinse it in cold water before using.	Removes potentially irritating disinfectant. Hot water might cause mercury to expand and break bulb.
4. Wipe thermometer from bulb end toward finger in a rotating manner. Dispose of tissue.	Rotating friction helps remove microorganisms. Wiping toward fingers prevents contamination of bulb end.
5. Read mercury level.	Mercury should be below 35.5° C (96° F) and below client's actual temperature before use.
6. If mercury is above desired level, shake thermometer down. Grasp upper end securely and stand away from any solid objects. Sharply flick wrist downward as though cracking a whip. Continue until reading is at appropriate level.	Brisk shaking lowers mercury level in glass tube. Standing in open spot prevents breakage of thermometer.
7. Assist client to a sitting or supine position.	Full access to axilla improves accuracy of temperature reading.
8. Draw curtains around bed and/or close room door.	Provides privacy and minimizes client embarrassment.

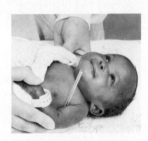

Fig. 2

Steps	Rationale
9. Move clothing or gown away from client's shoulder and arm.	Provides optimal exposure of axilla.
10. Insert thermometer into center of client's axilla, lower arm over thermometer, and place forearm across his chest. (Fig. 2)	Maintains proper position of thermometer against blood vessels in axilla.
11. Leave thermometer in place for 10 minutes or as long as recommended by agency. Gently hold a child's arm in place.	It takes longer to get reading with exposure to an external site. Movement can cause displacement of thermometer.
12. Carefully remove thermometer.	
13. Wipe off any secretions with soft tissue. Wipe in a rotating fashion from tip to bulb. Dispose of tissue.	Prevents contact of microorganisms with your hands. Tip is area of least contamination, bulb area of greatest contamination.
14. Read thermometer.	
15. Wash thermometer in lukewarm soapy water. Rinse in cold water and dry.	Mechanically removes organic material that can interfere with disinfectant action.
16. Store thermometer in its container after shaking it down again.	Proper storage prevents breakage.
17. Wash hands.	Reduces transmission of microorganisms.
18. Record temperature in proper chart or flow sheet. Signify axillary reading by capital A.	Vital signs should be recorded immediately after measurement. A prevents later confusion with oral or rectal measurements.

Nurse Alert

It may be necessary to gently hold the child's arm against his side.

Client Teaching

Instruct mothers of young children how to position and restrain the child properly. Also explain the importance of keeping the thermometer inserted at least 10 minutes.

Pediatric Considerations

Stay with the child throughout the procedure. The immaturity of a child's temperature regulation mechanisms can cause sudden changes in body temperature. A newborn's body temperature normally ranges between 35.5° and 37.5° C (96° and 99.5° F).

Geriatric Considerations

Disturbances in temperature regulation that normally occur with aging may cause the client to have a lower than normal body temperature.

Electronic Temperature Measurement

Electronic thermometers are now commonly used throughout various health care agencies. The device, consisting of a battery-powered display unit, thin wire cord, and temperature-sensitive probe, is capable of recording a client's body temperature in seconds. The electronic thermometer is not necessarily more accurate than a glass thermometer. The variables that alter temperature measurements (such as drinking hot or cold liquids) affect all types of thermometers. The advantages of the electronic thermometer are the quickness of recording and the safety from breakage and infection. Plastic probe covers protect clients when biting down during oral measurements and reduce cross-contamination between clients.

Potential Nursing Diagnoses

After assessing the client's temperature and observing for signs and symptoms of temperature alterations, the nurse may make the following nursing diagnosis:

   Potential for injury related to infection

Equipment

Electronic thermometer with probe
Probe cover
Lubricant (for rectal measurement)

Steps	Rationale
1. Wash hands.	Reduces transmission of microorganisms.
2. Close room door or bedside curtain.	Provides for client privacy.
3. Assist client to appropriate position for access to selected temperature site.	Ensures correct thermometer placement and accurate readings.
4. Choose correct temperature probe (usually color coded blue for oral or axillary and red for rectal) and connect to electronic display unit. (Fig. 3)	Separate probes prevent contamination of body cavities during use.

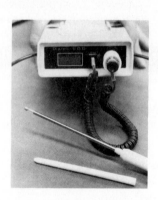

Fig. 3

5. Make sure that display window shows no temperature reading.	Will ensure proper registering of client's temperature.
6. Grasp probe at top, without pushing ejection button.	Ejection button ejects probe cover.
7. Place clean disposable plastic cover over temperature probe.	Prevents transmission of microorganisms between clients.

Steps	Rationale
8. Explain procedure to client.	Certain clients may be unfamiliar with measuring device. Explanation will relieve client anxiety.
9. Insert probe into selected body site, following same techniques as with mercury thermometers.	Ensures accurate readings. Correct techniques prevent injury to client.
10. Keep probe in place until electronic unit alarms and temperature reading appears on digital display.	Electronic units are capable of registering client's body temperature in seconds.
11. Note temperature reading.	
12. Gently remove probe and eject probe cover into trash receptacle by pushing ejection button.	Reduces spread of infection.
13. Replace probe in electronic unit.	Battery unit is rechargeable.
14. Help client return to desired comfortable position.	Maintains client's sense of well-being.
15. Wash your hands.	Reduces transmission of microorganisms.
16. Record temperature in vital signs flow sheet or nurse's notes.	Vital signs should be recorded immediately for accuracy.

Nurse Alert

Use whatever precautions are necessary to restrain the client or to hold the probe in place without injuring the client.

Client Teaching

Electronic thermometers are not used in the home setting. Thus explanation of the procedure is all that is necessary.

Pediatric Considerations

Carefully restrain a child to prevent the probe from injuring the oral or rectal tissues. Risk of injury is less than with glass thermometers. (Refer to previous temperature measurement skills.)

Geriatric Considerations

An elderly client may require assistance with positioning due to musculoskeletal disabilities. Remember, an elderly person's body temperature can normally be lower than that of a younger adult.

Assessing Radial Pulse

The character of a client's pulse provides valuable data regarding the integrity of his cardiovascular system.

The nurse commonly assesses the radial artery pulse during routine measurement of a client's vital signs or when a change is expected in his condition. The radial pulse is usually the most accessible. When it is inaccessible because of a dressing, cast, or other encumbrance, the apical pulse can be read instead. This involves auscultating heart sounds with a stethoscope placed medially below the left nipple.

Before assessing a client's pulse, the nurse attempts to control four factors—exercise, anxiety, pain, and postural change—that might cause false elevations or drops in heart rate. The nurse should also be able to anticipate how certain medications or disease processes will affect the client's heart rate.

Potential Nursing Diagnoses

After assessing the client's pulse, the nurse may make the following nursing diagnoses:

Alteration in cardiac output related to conduction or contractility deficit

Potential alteration in tissue perfusion related to arterial obstruction

Potential activity intolerance related to impaired cardiac output

Equipment

Wristwatch with second hand or digital display

Steps	Rationale
1. Wash hands.	Reduces chances of transmitting microorganisms.
2. Explain purpose and method of procedure to client.	Relieves client anxiety and facilitates his cooperation during procedure.
3. Have client assume a supine or sitting position. If supine, place his arm across his lower chest with wrist extended and palm down. (Fig. 4) If sitting, bend his elbow 90 degrees and support his lower arm on chair or on your arm. Extend his wrist with palm down.	Proper positioning fully exposes radial artery for palpation.

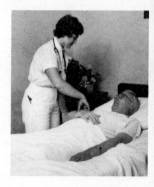

Fig. 4

4. Place tips of first three fingers of your hand along groove overlying radial artery and lightly compress against radius.	Fingertips are most sensitive to vibration. Do not palpate with thumb, or you may feel your own pulse accidentally.
5. Obliterate pulse initially and then relax pressure so pulse is easily palpable.	Pulse is most accurately assessed with moderate pressure. Too much pressure occludes it; too little prevents it from being felt with regularity.
6. When pulse can be felt regularly, use watch's second hand and begin to count rate, starting with zero, and then one, etc.	Rate is determined accurately only after assessor is assured that pulse can be palpated. Timing should begin with zero. Count of 1 is first beat felt after timing begins.

Steps	Rationale
7. If pulse is regular, count for 15 seconds and multiply total by 4.	Regular rate can be accurately assessed in 15 seconds.
8. If pulse is irregular, count for full minute.	Ensures accurate count.
9. Assess rhythm and strength of pulse (and elasticity of arterial wall).	Provides complete assessment of pulse character.
10. Assist client to comfortable position.	Promotes sense of well-being.
11. Record characteristics of pulse in medical record or flow sheet. Report abnormalities to nurse in charge or physician.	Provides data for monitoring changes in client's condition. Abnormalities may necessitate medical therapy.

Nurse Alert

If the nurse detects an irregular rhythm, it is important to assess for a pulse deficit. Compare the pulses at the radial artery and the apex of the heart. A difference between rates indicates a deficit.

Client Teaching

Certain clients should learn how to assess their own pulse. Those receiving medications that affect heart function should assess their pulse as well as any undesirable effects of medications. Clients undergoing cardiovascular and pulmonary rehabilitation should also assess their pulse to determine exercise tolerance.

Pediatric Considerations

An infant's heart rate at birth ranges from 100 to 160 beats per minute. By age 4 years the pulse rate slows to 80 to 120 beats per minute. With adolescence it varies between 60 and 100 beats per minute.

Geriatric Considerations

The normal range of an adult's pulse rate is 60 to 100 beats per minute. There should be no changes in an elderly client's heart rate at rest and in the absence of disease.

Assessing
Respirations

When the nurse assesses a client's respirations, the procedure involves observing the rate, depth, and rhythm of his ventilatory movements. She must be able to recognize normal passive breathing compared with ventilations that require muscular effort. Minimal effort is required to inhale and even less to exhale. If a client is having respiratory difficulties, the intercostal and accessory muscles will work more actively and the nurse will be able to see pronounced movement of his shoulder, neck, and chest muscles.

The nurse should be familiar with factors that normally affect respirations as well as conditions that place a client at risk of respiratory alterations.

Potential Nursing Diagnoses

After assessing a client's respirations, the nurse may make the following nursing diagnoses:

Ineffective airway clearance related to pain, position restrictions, or fatigue

Altered breathing pattern related to effects of analgesics, pain, or pulmonary infection

Equipment

Wristwatch with second hand or digital display

Steps	Rationale
1. Be sure that client is in comfortable position, preferably sitting.	Discomfort can cause client to breathe more rapidly.
2. Place client's arm in relaxed position across his abdomen or lower chest, or place your hand directly over client's upper abdomen.	This position is used during assessment of pulse. Both your and the client's hands rise and fall during respiratory cycle. Measuring respirations immediately after pulse assessment makes measurement inconspicuous.
3. Observe complete respiratory cycle (one inspiration and one expiration).	Ensures that count will begin with normal respiratory cycle.
4. Once a cycle is observed, look at watch's second hand and begin to count rate: when second hand hits number on dial, count ''one'' to begin first full cycle.	Timing begins with count of one. Respirations occur more slowly than pulse; thus count begins with one.
5. For an adult, count number of respirations in 30 seconds and multiply by 2. For infant or young child, count respirations for full minute.	Respiratory rate is equivalent to number of respirations per minute. Young infants and children breathe in an irregular rhythm.
6. If an adult's respirations have irregular rhythm or are abnormally slow or fast, count for full minute.	Accurate interpretation requires assessment for at least 1 minute.
7. While counting, note whether depth is shallow, normal, or deep and whether rhythm is normal or contains altered patterns.	The character of ventilatory movements may reveal specific alterations or disease states.
8. Record results in chart or flow sheet. Report any signs of respiratory alterations.	Provides data for monitoring change in client's condition. Abnormalities may indicate need for therapy.

Client Teaching

Clients with chronic lung disease can benefit from diaphragmatic breathing exercises (see Skill 8-1).

Pediatric Considerations

The nurse should plan on assessing respirations as the first vital sign in an infant or child. Startling or arousing an infant for other preliminary measurements can falsely increase respirations. Usually the nurse can simply observe respirations as the infant or young child lies in bed with his chest and abdomen uncovered.

A newborn breathes at a rate of 30 to 60 respirations per minute. A 2-year-old breathes 20 to 30 respirations per minute. A 6-year-old has a rate of 18 to 26 breaths per minute.

Geriatric Considerations

An adult normally breathes 12 to 20 respirations per minute at rest. With advancing age the average respiratory rate increases and chest expansion tends to decline due to increased rigidity of the chest wall.

Assessing Blood Pressure by Auscultation

For blood to flow throughout the circulatory system the heart pumps it into the arteries under high pressure. Pressure within the aorta at the time of left ventricular contraction (systole) is approximately 120 mm Hg in a healthy adult who is upright but not exercising. Once the aorta distends, a pressure wave traveling through the arterial system sends blood to the peripheral tissues. As the ventricles relax, pressure in the arterial system falls. The diastolic pressure (normally 80 mm Hg) is the minimal pressure exerted against the arterial walls. The nurse records blood pressure with the systolic before the diastolic reading (for example, 120/80).

The nurse's assessment of blood pressure helps determine the balance of several hemodynamic factors: cardiac output, peripheral vascular resistance, blood volume and viscosity, elasticity of the arteries. A client's blood pressure should be carefully compared with pulse rate and character in addition to other cardiovascular assessment findings so an intelligent conclusion can be drawn regarding the client's circulatory status.

Potential Nursing Diagnoses

After assessing the client's blood pressure and reviewing other cardiovascular findings, the nurse may make the following nursing diagnoses:

Alteration in cardiac output

Alteration in cardiopulmonary and peripheral tissue perfusion

Equipment

Stethoscope
Sphygmomanometer with cuff

Steps	Rationale
1. Determine proper cuff size. Width of inflatable bladder within cuff should be 40% of circumference at midpoint of limb on which cuff is to be used (or 20% wider than diameter). Length of bladder should be about twice recommended width.	Proper cuff size is necessary so correct amount of pressure is applied over artery. Cuffs that are too narrow, too wide, or improperly applied cause false-high or false-low readings.
2. Wash hands.	Reduces transmission of microorganisms.
3. Explain to client purpose of procedure.	Reassures client.
4. Assist client to comfortable sitting position, with arm slightly flexed, forearm supported at heart level, and palm turned up.	Having arm above heart level would produce false-low readings. This position facilitates cuff application.
5. Expose client's upper arm fully.	Ensures proper cuff application.
6. Palpate brachial artery (on lower medial side of biceps muscle). Position cuff 2.5 cm (1 inch) above site of pulsations (antecubital fossa). (Fig. 5)	Stethoscope will be placed over artery without touching cuff.
7. Center arrows marked on cuff along brachial artery.	Inflating bladder directly over brachial artery ensures that proper pressure is applied during inflation.

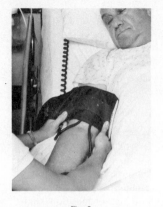

Fig. 5

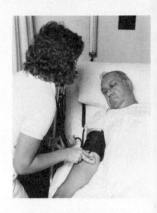

Fig. 6

Steps	Rationale
8. Be sure that cuff is fully deflated. Wrap cuff evenly and snugly around upper arm.	Ensures that proper pressure will be applied over artery.
9. Be sure that manometer is positioned at eye level.	Ensures accurate reading of mercury level.
10. If you do not know client's normal systolic pressure, palpate radial artery and inflate cuff to 30 mm Hg above pressure at which radial pulsation disappears. Deflate cuff and wait 30 seconds.	Determines maximal inflation point and prevents auscultatory gap. The 30-second delay prevents venous congestion and falsely high readings.
11. Place stethoscope earpieces in your ears and be sure sounds are clear, not muffled.	Each earpiece should follow angle of your ear canal to facilitate hearing.
12. Relocate brachial artery and place diaphragm (or bell) of stethoscope over it. (Fig. 6)	Ensures optimal sound reception. American Heart Association recommends use of bell for detecting low-pitched Korotkoff sounds.

Steps	Rationale
13. Close valve of pressure bulb clockwise until tight.	Prevents air leak during inflation.
14. Inflate cuff to 30 mm Hg above client's normal systolic level.	Ensures accurate pressure measurement.
15. Slowly release valve, allowing mercury to fall at rate of 2-3 mm Hg per second.	Too rapid or too slow decline in mercury level may lead to inaccurate reading.
16. Note point on manometer at which first clear sound is heard.	First Korotkoff sound indicates systolic pressure.
17. Continue to deflate cuff gradually, noting point at which sound becomes muffled or dampened.	Fourth Korotkoff sound may be detected as diastolic pressure in adults with hypertension. American Heart Association recommends it as indication of diastolic pressure in children.
18. Continue cuff deflation and note point at which sound disappears.	American Heart Association recommends recording fifth Korotkoff sound as diastolic pressure in adults.
19. Deflate cuff rapidly and remove it from client's arm unless you need to repeat measurement.	Continuous inflation causes arterial occlusion, resulting in numbness and tingling (paresthesia) of client's arm.
20. If repeating procedure, wait 30 seconds.	Prevents venous congestion and falsely high readings.
21. Fold cuff and store it properly.	Proper maintenance of supplies contributes to instrument accuracy.
22. Assist client to position he prefers and cover his upper arm.	Maintains client's comfort.
23. Record findings on medical record or flow sheet.	Should be done immediately.

Nurse Alert

Be aware of signs and symptoms of high blood pressure (hypertension): headache (usually occipital), flushing of the face, nosebleed, fatigue in elderly clients. Be aware also of the signs and symptoms of low blood pressure (hypotension): dizziness, mental confusion, restlessness, pale or cyanotic (dusky) skin and mucous membranes, cool mottled skin over the extremities.

Client Teaching

Clients should understand the risk factors of high blood pressure: obesity, increased sodium intake, increased cholesterol intake, smoking, lack of exercise. When clients are taking antihypertensive medications, review their medication schedules and assess their understanding of the purpose and importance of the medication.

Pediatric Considerations

A newborn (3000 g or 6.6 pounds) has an average systolic pressure of 50 to 52, diastolic of 25 to 30, and mean of 35 to 40 mm Hg. At 4 years the average blood pressure is 85/60; at 6 years it averages 95/62; and at 12 years, 108/67.

Geriatric Considerations

With aging there is a reduction in blood vessel compliance and an increase in peripheral resistance to blood flow. Arteriosclerosis is a common disorder with advancing age, although it can begin early in adulthood. Because of vascular changes, elderly clients are at risk of significantly increased systolic and slightly increased diastolic pressures.

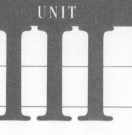

POSITIONING
AND
TRANSFER

UNIT

III

Proper Lifting

The nurse must use proper lifting techniques to reduce the risk of injuring her musculoskeletal system and to decrease the risk of hurting the client. Before lifting, she must determine that the object to be lifted is in the right position, at the right height, and less than or equal to the maximum weight that she can safely lift. In addition, she must determine that her own body is correctly positioned for safe lifting.

Potential Nursing Diagnoses

Clients for whom proper lifting techniques may be required can have one or more of the following nursing diagnoses:

Impaired physical mobility related to fatigue, trauma, or decreased level of consciousness

Self-care deficit related to restricted mobility

Potential for injury related to improper lifting

Steps	Rationale
1. Assess "basic four" lifting measures: position of object, height of object, body position, and maximum weight.	Determines need for assistance from additional personnel during lift.
2. Come close to object to be moved.	Increases your body balance during lift.
3. Enlarge your base of support, placing feet apart.	Maintains better body balance, reducing your risk of falling.

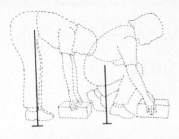

Fig. 7

Steps	Rationale
4. Lower your center of gravity to object to be lifted. Flex at knees and hips. (Fig. 7)	Increases body balance and enables your muscle groups to work together in synchronized manner.
5. Maintain proper alignment of head and neck with vertebrae.	Reduces risk of injuring your lumbar vertebrae and muscle groups.

Nurse Alert

Before lifting an object, the nurse should decide if she will be able to safely lift it alone. If she feels that she cannot (the object is too large or too heavy), she should seek additional personnel to help her.

Client Teaching

Demonstrating correct lifting techniques is an excellent way for the nurse to teach the client and family how they can avoid injuring themselves when moving something.

Geriatric Considerations

The geriatric client may require re-education on what he can and cannot safely lift. Objects that could be safely lifted in the middle and late adult years cannot usually be lifted in the later adult years.

Ensuring Proper Positioning

Correct positioning of a client is crucial for maintaining proper body alignment. Any client with decreased mobility is at risk of developing contractures, postural abnormalities, and pressure sores. The nurse has the primary responsibility to minimize this risk, which is done by changing an immobilized client's position at least every 2 hours.

Potential Nursing Diagnoses

Clients who require positioning may have one or more of the following nursing diagnoses:

Impaired mobility related to casted extremity or to paralysis

Potential impairment of skin integrity related to limited mobility

Alteration in peripheral tissue perfusion related to limited mobility

Steps	Rationale
1. Wash hands.	Reduces transfer of microorganisms.
2. Raise level of bed to comfortable working height.	Elevates level of work toward your center of gravity.
3. Determine what equipment is needed. Organize work area. Remove obstacles.	Provides for safe organized positioning.

Steps	Rationale
4. Tell client what you are doing and what he can do to help.	Enables you to use client's mobility and strength, if possible.
5. Determine if you will need assistance and get it before beginning to change client's position.	Gives you an opportunity to assess your ability to move client independently and ensures your safety as well as that of client.
6. Place one pillow beneath client's head.	Provides support to head without causing flexion, hyperextension, or lateral flexion of neck.
7. Determine that client's elbows, knees, and hips are supported and slightly flexed.	Ensures proper alignment when these joints are supported. Flexion prevents prolonged hyperextension, which could impair joint mobility.
8. Determine that client's feet are supported. If he is in bed, provide footboard or sandbags, if necessary. If in chair or wheelchair, position his feet flat on floor, on footrest of wheelchair, or on another support device.	Support maintains dorsal flexion and helps prevent footdrop.
9. Determine that his extremities are supported and, whenever possible, in positions for free movement.	Reduces risk of joint dislocation, particularly when there is underlying nerve damage (as after stroke). Allowing extremity to move freely helps maintain joint mobility.
10. Check that any bony prominences are not permitted to remain in direct contact with other parts of his body (e.g., knee resting on thigh of other leg in side-lying position).	Pressure increases risk of skin breakdown and damage to musculoskeletal system.

Steps	Rationale
11. Change his body position at least every 2 hours.	Removes pressure from dependent body tissues, lessening risk of venous pooling.
12. Massage pressure areas after each position change.	Increases blood supply to pressure areas and reduces risk of pressure sores.
13. Wash your hands.	Reduces transmission of microorganisms.
14. Record in nurse's notes client's new position.	Documents that procedure was performed.

Nurse Alert

When positioning clients, the nurse must be aware of the fact that certain traumatic or postoperative conditions require the client to be placed in specific positions. For example, a supine position may be necessary for clients after some spinal surgery.

Client Teaching

Teach the client which position or positions are appropriate to decrease stress on his musculoskeletal system and to promote optimal relaxation.

Pediatric Considerations

The pediatric client usually requires positioning to maintain alignment of a fractured extremity or to prevent accidental removal of a tube or drain. Nursing measures must be designed to safely restrain the young child as well as prevent him from changing positions.

Geriatric Considerations

An elderly client is at greater risk than a younger client of skin breakdown or joint deformities related to immobility. Therefore his nursing care plan may require more frequent position changes, such as every hour or every 90 minutes instead of every 2 hours.

Supported Fowler
Position

The supported Fowler position improves cardiac output and ventilation as well as facilitates urinary and bowel elimination. In this position the head of the client's bed is raised 45 to 60 degrees and the client's knees are slightly elevated so there will be no restriction of circulation to the lower extremities. Proper alignment of the body when the client is in this position requires support that maintains comfort and reduces the risk of damage to body systems.

Potential Nursing Diagnoses

Clients placed in the supported Fowler position may have one or more of the following nursing diagnoses:

Potential impairment of skin integrity related to improper positioning

Altered tissue perfusion related to immobility

Ineffective breathing pattern related to positioning

Steps	Rationale
1. Wash hands.	Reduces transmission of microorganisms.
2. Position client supine with his head near headboard.	Prevents client from sliding toward foot of bed when head of bed is elevated.
3. Raise head of bed 45-60 degrees.	Increases client comfort, improves breathing, and increases his opportunity to socialize, relax, or watch television.

Steps	Rationale
4. Allow client's head to rest against mattress or on very small pillow.	Prevents flexion contracture of client's cervical vertebrae.
5. If large pillow is used, turn it lengthwise to support client's upper back, shoulders, and head.	Prevents flexion contracture of his cervical vertebrae and maintains vertebral alignment.
6. Use pillows to support client's arms and hands if he does not have voluntary control or use of upper extremities.	Prevents shoulder dislocation from downward gravitational pull of unsupported arms, promotes circulation by preventing venous pooling, reduces edema in hands or arms, and prevents flexion contractures of wrist.
7. Position pillow at client's lower back.	Supports lumbar vertebrae and decreases spinal flexion.
8. Place small pillow or roll under client's thighs. If his lower extremities are paralyzed or he is unable to control lower extremities, use a roll under his trochanters in addition to a pillow under his thighs. (Fig. 8)	Prevents hyperextension of knees and occlusion of popliteal artery due to pressure from body weight. Trochanter roll prevents external rotation of legs.
9. Place small pillow or roll under client's ankle region.	Eliminates prolonged pressure from bed on heels.
10. Place footboard at bottom of his feet.	Maintains dorsal flexion and prevents foot-drop.

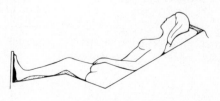

Fig. 8

Steps	Rationale
11. Wash your hands.	Reduces transmission of microorganisms.
12. Record in nurse's notes client's new position.	Documents that procedure was performed.

Nurse Alert

Clients in the Fowler position are at risk of cervical flexion contractures if the pillow is too thick. Additional complications may include external rotation of the hips, foot-drop, and skin breakdown at the sacrum and heels.

Client Teaching

The Fowler position provides an excellent opportunity for the nurse to implement client teaching in self-care (as with the newly diagnosed diabetic client), skin care, and knowledge about medications.

Geriatric Considerations

Elderly clients are at greater risk than younger clients of skin breakdown due to increased capillary fragility, decreased muscle mass, and reduced skin moisture.

Supported Supine Position

The supine position, also called the dorsal recumbent position, may be required after spinal surgery and the administration of some spinal anesthetics. In this position the relationship of body parts is essentially the same as in proper standing alignment except that the body is horizontal.

Potential Nursing Diagnoses

Clients placed supine may have one or more of the following nursing diagnoses:

Potential impairment of skin integrity related to improper positioning

Altered tissue perfusion related to immobility

Potential self-care deficit for feeding, hygiene, grooming, and toileting related to supine position

Steps	Rationale
1. Wash hands.	Reduces transmission of microorganisms.
2. Place client flat in center of bed.	Prepares client for proper positioning.
3. Place pillow under client's shoulders, neck, and head, unless contraindicated following some spinal surgery or anesthetic administration.	Maintains correct alignment and prevents flexion contracture as well as hyperextension of cervical vertebrae.

Steps	Rationale
4. Place small pillow or roll under client's lumbar spine. (Fig. 9)	Provides support to lumbar vertebrae, especially when firm mattress is being used, and reduces flexion of lumbar vertebrae.
5. When necessary, place rolls under client's trochanters or sandbags parallel with lateral surface of his thighs.	Reduces external rotation of the legs.
6. Place small pillow or roll under his upper legs to flex knees slightly.	Prevents hyperextension of knees and improves circulation by reducing pressure from bed on the popliteal artery.
7. Place small pillow or roll under client's ankles to elevate heels.	Raising heels from surface of bed reduces pressure on them.
8. Place footboard against bottom of client's feet.	Maintains dorsal flexion and prevents foot-drop.
9. Place pillows under client's forearms, maintaining upper arms parallel with his body. (Fig. 10)	Reduces internal rotation of shoulders and prevents extension of elbows.

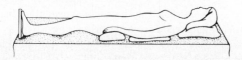

Fig. 9

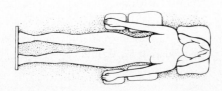

Fig. 10

Steps	Rationale
10. Have client grasp hand rolls or towels or use hand splints when available.	Reduces extension of fingers and abduction of thumb. Also maintains thumb slightly adducted and in opposition to the fingers.
11. Wash your hands.	Reduces transmission of microorganisms.
12. Record in nurse's notes client's new position.	Documents that procedure was performed.

Nurse Alert

Clients in the supine position are at risk of internal rotation of the shoulders, external rotation of the hips, foot-drop, and pressure sores at the lumbar vertebrae, elbows, heels, and scapulas.

Client Teaching

While the client is supine, the nurse can teach him and his family the prescribed range of joint motion exercises and skin care measures.

Pediatric Considerations

A child may be restrained in the supine position to maintain patency of an intravenous catheter or the integrity of postoperative drains. The nurse should incorporate into her plan of care time to hold and play with the child.

Geriatric Considerations

Elderly clients are at greater risk than younger clients of skin breakdown due to increased capillary fragility, decreased muscle mass, and reduced skin moisture.

Supported Prone
Position

The primary therapeutic use of the prone position is to provide an alternative for clients who are immobilized or on prolonged bedrest. It is not a well-tolerated position, and frequent changes are required to relieve boredom and discomfort.

Potential Nursing Diagnoses

Clients who must be maintained prone may have one or more of the following nursing diagnoses:

> Impaired physical mobility related to fatigue or decreased level of consciousness
>
> Diversional activities deficit related to limitations of position
>
> Self-care deficit: feeding, hygiene, grooming, and toileting, related to restricted mobility
>
> Potential for injury related to risk of aspiration

Steps	Rationale
1. Wash hands.	Reduces transmission of microorganisms.
2. Place client on his abdomen in center of bed.	Prepares client for proper positioning.
3. Turn client's head to one side and support with small pillow. When excessive drainage from mouth is present, pillow may be contraindicated. (Fig. 11)	Reduces flexion or hyperextension of cervical vertebrae.

Steps	Rationale
4. Place small pillow under client's belly below level of diaphragm.	Reduces pressure on breasts in some female clients, decreases hyperextension of lumbar vertebrae, and improves breathing by reducing pressure on diaphragm from mattress.
5. Position client toward foot of bed so his feet hang over mattress, or support lower legs with pillow to elevate toes. (Fig. 12)	Prevents foot-drop and reduces external rotation of legs and pressure on toes from mattress.
6. Wash your hands.	Reduces transmission of microorganisms.
7. Record in nurse's notes client's new position.	Documents that procedure was performed.

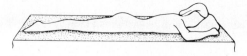

Fig. 11

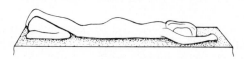

Fig. 12

Nurse Alert

When placing a client in the prone position, the nurse should be sure that a pillow is under the client's lower legs to promote dorsiflexion of the ankles and knee flexion. Body alignment is poor when the ankles are continuously in plantar flexion and the lumbar spine remains hyperextended. In addition, the nurse must frequently assess the client's breathing patterns to detect any alterations that might result from the prone position.

Client Teaching

When the client is prone, the nurse can effectively teach his family about skin care or any dressing changes on the back that may be required.

Pediatric Considerations

Children placed prone usually do not tolerate the position well because of limited eye contact with their environment. When the prone position is required, the nurse should incorporate quiet play or stories into her plan of care.

Geriatric Considerations

Elderly clients may become disoriented when in the prone position because of decreased visual cues from their environment. The nurse can reduce this risk by placing a clock within the client's visual field, increasing the amount of time she spends with the client, and encouraging visitation by family.

Supported Side-Lying (Lateral) Position

The side-lying position removes pressure from any bony prominences on the client's back and redistributes the major portion of his body weight on the dependent hip and shoulder. In this position the client's trunk alignment should be the same as in proper standing posture.

Potential Nursing Diagnoses

Clients in the side-lying (lateral) position may have one or more of the following nursing diagnoses:

Impaired physical mobility related to fatigue or decreased level of consciousness

Deficit in diversional activities related to limitations of prone position

Self-care deficit: feeding, hygiene, grooming, and toileting, related to restricted mobility

Potential for injury related to risk of aspiration

Steps	Rationale
1. Wash hands.	Reduces transmission of microorganisms.
2. Place client supine in center of bed.	Aligns client properly.
3. Roll client onto his side.	Prepares him for proper positioning.

Steps	Rationale
4. Place pillow under client's head and neck.	Maintains alignment, reduces lateral flexion of neck, and decreases muscle strain on major neck muscle (sternocleidomastoid).
5. Both his arms should be slightly flexed: upper arm supported by a pillow under the forearm, lower arm supported by the mattress.	Decreases internal rotation and adduction of shoulder, preventing dislocation. Supporting both arms in a slightly flexed position protects joints and improves ventilation because chest is able to expand more easily.
6. Place one or two pillows under client's upper leg. Pillows should support leg evenly from groin to foot. (Figs. 13, 14, 15)	Prevents internal rotation and adduction of thigh and reduces pressure to bony prominences of leg from mattress.
7. Place supports, such as sandbags and footboard, at client's feet as needed.	Prevents foot-drop.
8. Place rolled pillow parallel with his back.	Maintains support and alignment of vertebrae. Also keeps client from rolling back out of alignment and prevents rotation of spine.

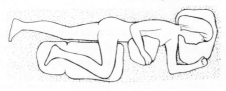

Fig. 13

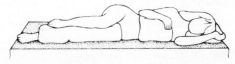

Fig. 14

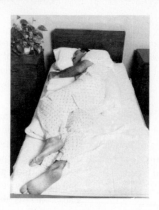

Fig. 15

Steps	Rationale
9. Wash your hands.	Reduces transmission of microorganisms.
10. Record in nurse's notes client's new position.	Documents that procedure was performed.

Nurse Alert

When placing a client in the side-lying position, the nurse should use caution to avoid lateral flexion of the neck, improper spinal alignment, internal rotation of the hips and shoulder joints, foot-drop, and pressure on the ilium, knees, and ankles.

Client Teaching

The side-lying position provides the nurse an excellent opportunity to teach the client (and family) about therapeutic measures that may be continued in the home.

Pediatric Considerations

The side-lying position is used with an unconscious, immobilized, or burned child. If the child is alert, the nurse should incorporate quiet diversional activities into her care plan so this position will be maintained.

Geriatric Considerations

Elderly clients are at greater risk than younger clients of skin breakdown caused by increased capillary fragility, decreased muscle mass, and reduced skin moisture.

Supported Sims (Semiprone) Position

The Sims position is frequently used for an unconscious client to increase drainage of mucus from the mouth. In addition, it provides an alternative for clients who are immobilized or on bedrest. In this position the client's weight is placed on the anterior ilium and the humerus and clavicle.

Potential Nursing Diagnoses

Clients placed in the Sims position may have one or more of the following nursing diagnoses:

Potential impairment of skin integrity related to immobility

Altered tissue perfusion related to immobility

Potential self-care deficit for feeding, hygiene, grooming, and toileting related to restricted mobility

Impaired physical mobility related to fatigue or decreased level of consciousness

Steps	Rationale
1. Wash hands.	Reduces transmission of microorganisms.
2. Place client on his abdomen in center of bed.	Prepares client for proper positioning.
3. Turn client's head to side and place small pillow underneath.	Maintains proper alignment and prevents lateral flexion of neck.
4. Place a pillow under client's flexed arm. Pillow should extend from his hand to elbow. (Figs. 16, 17)	Prevents internal rotation of shoulder.

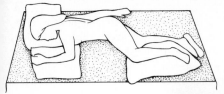

Fig. 16

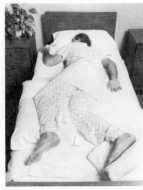

Fig. 17

Steps	Rationale
5. Place another pillow under his flexed leg, to extend from knee to foot.	Prevents internal rotation of hip and adduction of leg. Also reduces pressure on knees and ankles from mattress.
6. Place sandbags parallel to plantar surface of client's foot.	Prevents foot-drop.
7. Wash your hands.	Reduces transmission of microorganisms.
8. Record in nurse's notes client's new position.	Documents that procedure was performed.

Nurse Alert

The nurse should be aware of potential trouble areas with the Sims position: lateral flexion of the neck; internal rotation, adduction, or lack of support to the shoulders and hips; footdrop; and potential pressure sores at the ears, ilium, humerus, clavicle, knees, and ankles.

Client Teaching

The Sims position provides the nurse an opportunity to teach the family about range of joint motion and skin care. In addition, the nurse can demonstrate proper positioning measures.

Pediatric Considerations

The Sims position is used with an unconscious, immobilized, or burned child. If the child is alert, the nurse should incorporate quiet diversional activities into her care plan so the Sims position will be maintained.

Geriatric Considerations

Because of the normal aging process, an elderly client's musculoskeletal system is at risk of joint deformities, loss of muscle mass, and skin breakdown. If degenerative joint disease (osteoarthritis) is also present, the client may require his position to be changed every hour instead of every 2 hours.

Assisting a Client to Move Up in Bed (One or Two Nurses)

The nurse will frequently encounter a semi-helpless, helpless, or immobilized client whose position must be changed or who must be moved up in bed. Proper use of body mechanics can enable her (and a helper) to move, lift, or transfer such a client safely and at the same time avoid musculoskeletal injury.

Potential Nursing Diagnoses

Clients requiring assistance to move up in bed may have one or more of the following nursing diagnoses:

Potential for impaired activity tolerance related to fatigue or restricted mobility

Potential for impaired skin integrity related to restricted mobility or pressure

Impaired physical mobility related to fatigue or decreased level of consciousness

Steps	Rationale
1. Wash hands.	Reduces transmission of microorganisms.
2. Face head of bed. (If two nurses are assisting client, each stands at one side of bed.)	Facing direction of movement prevents twisting of your body when moving client.

97

Steps	Rationale
3. Place your feet apart with foot nearer bed behind other foot.	Increases your balance. One foot behind other allows you to transfer your body weight as client is moved up in bed.
4. If possible, ask client to flex his knees, bringing his feet as close to buttocks as possible.	Enables client to use his leg muscles during process of actually moving up in bed.
5. Instruct client to flex his neck, tilting chin toward chest.	Prevents hyperextension of neck when moving to head of bed.
6. Ask him to assist in moving by using trapeze bar if available or pushing on bed surface.	He uses his upper extremity muscles to elevate trunk and reduce friction when moving up in bed.
7. If client has limited upper extremity strength or mobility, place his arms across his chest.	Prevents friction from arms dragging across bed surface during move.
8. Flex your knees and hips, bringing your forearms closer to level of bed.	Increases your balance and strength by bringing your center of gravity closer to client, the "object" to be moved.
9. Place arm that is closer to head of bed under client's shoulder and other arm under client's thighs.	Prevents trauma to client's musculoskeletal system, because his shoulder and hip joints are supported. Also evenly distributes client's weight.
10. Instruct client to move up in bed on count of three.	Prepares client for actual move, thus reinforcing his assistance.
11. On count of three, rock and shift your weight from back leg to front leg. At same time, have client push with his heels and elevate his trunk. (Fig. 18)	Enables you to improve your balance and overcome inertia. Shifting your weight counteracts client's weight. When client pushes with his heels and lifts his trunk, friction is reduced.

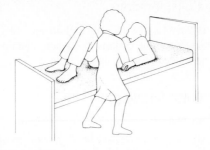

Fig. 18

Steps	Rationale
12. Reassess client's body alignment and pressure point areas. If poor, use nursing interventions to reduce risk of damage to your musculoskeletal system.	Proper body alignment increases client's comfort, promotes rest, and reduces hazards of immobility.
13. Record in nurse's notes client's new position.	Documents that procedure was performed.

Nurse Alert

The nurse must avoid dragging a client up in bed. Dragging against the bed linen causes shearing force. With a shearing force the skin adheres to the surface of the bed while the layers of subcutaneous tissue and even the bones slide in the direction of body movement. The underlying tissue capillaries are compressed and may be severed by the pressure.

Client Teaching

This skill provides an excellent opportunity for the nurse to teach a client and his family how to maintain proper body alignment while moving him up in bed.

Pediatric Considerations

The nurse is usually able to pick a child up and reposition him. However, when the child is in traction, additional assistance may be needed to maintain alignment.

Geriatric Considerations

Elderly clients with degenerative joint disease (osteoarthritis) are at greater risk than younger clients of shoulder joint dislocation while being moved. In addition, their decreased muscle mass and reduced skin elasticity and skin moisture increase their risk of skin breakdown from shearing force.

Moving a Helpless Client Up in Bed (One Nurse)

The nurse will frequently encounter a semi-helpless, helpless, or immobilized client whose position must be changed or who must be moved up in bed. Proper use of body mechanics can enable her to move, lift, or transfer such a client safely and also protect herself from musculoskeletal injury.

Potential Nursing Diagnoses

Clients requiring assistance to move up in bed may have one or more of the following nursing diagnoses:

Potential for impaired activity tolerance related to fatigue or restricted mobility

Potential for impaired skin integrity related to restricted mobility or pressure

Impaired physical mobility related to fatigue or decreased level of consciousness

Steps	Rationale
1. Place client in supine position with head of bed flat and all pillows removed. Stand on one side of bed.	Maintains client in supine position and enables you to easily assess his body alignment throughout move and to administer any additional care (e.g., suctioning or hygiene needs) during procedure. Lowering head of bed to flat position reduces gravitational pull on client's upper body. Removing all pillows from bed reduces interference from equipment during procedure.

Steps	Rationale
2. Begin at client's feet. Face foot of bed at 45-degree angle and slide client's legs diagonally toward head of bed.	Positioning is begun at client's legs because they are least weight to be supported. Facing direction of movement ensures proper balance for you. Diagonal motion permits pull in direction of move.
3. Move parallel with client's hips and flex your knees and hips as needed to bring your arms level with client's hips.	Maintains your proper alignment, brings you closest to "object" to be moved, and lowers your center of gravity as necessary.
4. Slide client's hips diagonally toward head of the bed. If available, a pull sheet may be useful. (A pull sheet is usually a full-sized bath blanket or sheet that is folded to extend the distance from client's shoulders to 2 inches below popliteal space. When moving client, use sheet to pull him or a portion of his body.)	Aligns client's hips and feet.
5. Move parallel with client's head and shoulders, flexing your knees and hips as necessary to bring your arms level with client's body.	Maintains your proper alignment, brings you closer to "object" to be moved, and lowers your center of gravity as necessary.
6. Slide arm closer to head of bed under client's head and neck, with your hand reaching under and supporting client's far shoulder.	Supports client's head and neck, maintaining their proper alignment during transfer. Placement of your hand on client's far shoulder supports that joint during move.

Steps	Rationale
7. Place your other arm under client's chest.	Supports client's body weight and reduces friction during movement.
8. Slide client's trunk, shoulders, head, and neck diagonally toward head of bed.	Realigns body on one side of bed.
9. Elevate side rail next to client. Move to other side and elevate side rail, switching sides of bed until client is at desired height.	Protects client from falling out of bed while being moved up.
10. Center client in bed, moving his body in same three sections.	Protects client from falling and provides ample room on either side of client for turning, positioning, or other nursing care activities.
11. Reassess client's body alignment and pressure point areas. If poor body alignment or pressure points are present, use nursing interventions to reduce risk of damage to his musculoskeletal system.	Proper body alignment increases client comfort, promotes rest, and reduces hazards of immobility.
12. Record in nurse's notes client's position in bed.	Documents that procedure was performed.

Nurse Alert

The nurse must avoid dragging a client up in bed. Dragging against the bed linen causes shearing force. With a shearing force the skin adheres to the surface of the bed while the layers of subcutaneous tissue and even the bones slide in the direction of body movement. The underlying tissue capillaries are compressed and may be severed by the pressure.

Client Teaching

This skill provides an excellent opportunity for the nurse to teach a client and his family how to maintain body alignment while moving him up in bed.

Pediatric Considerations

The nurse is usually able to pick a child up and reposition him. However, when the child is in traction, additional assistance may be needed to maintain alignment.

Geriatric Considerations

Elderly clients with degenerative joint disease (osteoarthritis) are at greater risk than younger clients of shoulder joint dislocation while being moved. In addition, their decreased muscle mass and reduced skin elasticity and skin moisture increase their risk of skin breakdown from shearing force.

Repositioning a Helpless Client

The nurse will frequently encounter a semi-helpless, helpless, or immobilized client whose position must be changed or who must be moved up in bed. Proper use of body mechanics can enable her to move, lift, or transfer such a client safely while at the same time protecting herself from musculoskeletal injury.

Potential Nursing Diagnoses

Clients requiring assistance to move up in bed may have one or more of the following nursing diagnoses:

Potential for impaired activity intolerance related to fatigue or restricted mobility

Potential for impaired skin integrity related to restricted mobility or pressure

Impaired physical mobility related to fatigue or decreased level of consciousness

Steps	Rationale
1. Wash hands.	Reduces transfer of microorganisms.
2. Lower head of bed, if elevated, to flat position.	Reduces gravitational pull on client's upper body.
▪ Remove all pillows and devices used in previous position.	Reduces interference during repositioning.
3. Face client, move close to bed, and assume a broad	Prevents twisting of your body, brings your center of

Steps	Rationale
stance with one foot in front of other.	gravity close to "object" being moved, and increases your balance.
4. Place your upper arm under client's shoulders while supporting his cervical vertebrae and head.	Supports alignment of client's shoulders and prevents flexion or hyperextension of his head and neck during repositioning.
5. Place your other arm under client's thighs.	Supports alignment of client's hips and evenly distributes his body weight.
6. Rock in direction of movement (i.e., if turning client to side, rock away from bed; if moving client toward center, rock toward bed).	Overcomes inertia and throws your body weight in direction of movement.
7. Assess client's skin for any reddened pressure points from previous position.	Early identification reduces risk of formation of pressure sores.
8. Massage pressure points.	Increases circulation to tissues and muscles.
9. Place client in supine, prone, side-lying, or Sims position (see Skills 3-4 to 3-7) and evaluate for proper alignment.	Rotation of positions reduces risk of damage to client's musculoskeletal system from immobility.
10. Record in nurse's notes client's new position.	Documents that procedure was performed.

Nurse Alert

The nurse must avoid dragging a client up in bed. Dragging against the bed linen causes shearing force. With a shearing force the skin adheres to the surface of the bed while the layers of subcutaneous tissue and even the bones slide in the direction of body movement. The underlying tissue capillaries are compressed and may be severed by the pressure.

Client Teaching

This skill provides an excellent opportunity for the nurse to teach a client and his family how to maintain body alignment while moving him up in bed.

Pediatric Considerations

The nurse is usually able to pick a child up and reposition him. However, when the child is in traction, additional assistance may be needed to maintain alignment.

Geriatric Considerations

Elderly clients with degenerative joint disease (osteoarthritis) are at greater risk than younger clients of shoulder joint dislocation while being moved. In addition, their decreased muscle mass and reduced skin elasticity and skin moisture increase the risk of skin breakdown from shearing force.

Assisting a Client
to the Sitting Position

A partially immobilized or weak client will require nursing assistance to sit up in bed. The nurse can help such a client attain the sitting position while maintaining proper body alignment for herself as well as the client. Correct positioning techniques will reduce the risk of musculoskeletal injury to all persons involved.

Potential Nursing Diagnoses

Clients requiring assistance to a sitting position may have one or more of the following nursing diagnoses:

Potential activity intolerance related to partial immobility or fatigue.

Potential impairment of skin integrity related to shearing force

Impaired physical mobility related to fatigue

Steps	Rationale
1. Place client in supine position.	Enables you to continually assess client's body alignment and administer additional care, such as suctioning or hygiene needs.
2. Remove all pillows.	Decreases interference while sitting client up in bed.
3. Face head of bed.	Reduces twisting of your body when moving client.
4. Place your feet apart with foot nearer bed behind other foot.	Improves your balance and allows you to transfer your body weight as client is moved to sitting position.

Steps	Rationale
5. Place hand that is farther from client under client's shoulders, supporting his head and cervical vertebrae.	Maintains alignment of client's head and cervical vertebrae and allows for even lifting of his upper trunk.
6. Place your other hand on bed surface.	Provides support and balance.
7. Raise client to a sitting position by shifting your weight from front leg to back leg. (Fig. 19)	Improves your balance, overcomes inertia, and transfers your weight in direction of move.
8. Push against bed and the arm that was on bed surface.	Divides activity of raising client to a sitting position between your arms and legs and protects your back from strain. By bracing one hand against mattress and pushing against it as you lift client, you transfer part of weight that would be lifted by your back muscles through your arms and onto mattress (Bilger and Greene, 1973).
9. Record in nurse's notes client's new position.	Documents that procedure was performed.

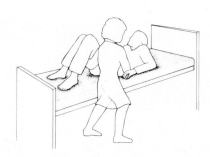

Fig. 19

Nurse Alert

The nurse must avoid dragging a client up in bed. Dragging against the bed linen causes shearing force. In addition, she should carefully observe the client for signs of the possible development of postural hypotension (dizziness, fainting, etc.).

Client Teaching

This skill provides an opportunity for the client and family to learn appropriate body alignment for the sitting position.

Pediatric Considerations

Children are usually easy to move, and the nurse may be able to simply raise a child to the sitting position.

Geriatric Considerations

Elderly clients with degenerative joint disease (osteoarthritis) are at greater risk than younger clients of shoulder joint dislocation while being moved. In addition, their decreased muscle mass and reduced skin elasticity and skin moisture increase the risk of skin breakdown from shearing force.

Assisting a Client to the Sitting Position on Side of Bed

The partially immobilized or weak client will require nursing assistance to attain a sitting position in bed. The nurse can help such a client sit up while at the same time maintaining proper body alignment for herself and the client and reducing the risk of musculoskeletal injuries to all persons involved. Frequently this is the first activity ordered for a client who has been on bedrest.

Potential Nursing Diagnosis

Clients requiring assistance to a sitting position on the side of the bed may have one or more of the following nursing diagnoses:

Potential activity intolerance related to partial immobility or fatigue

Potential impairment of skin integrity related to shearing force

Impaired physical mobility related to fatigue

Steps	Rationale
1. Place client in side-lying position, facing you on side of bed where he will be sitting. Put up side rail on opposite side.	Prepares client for move and protects him from falling.

Steps	Rationale
2. Raise head of bed to highest level (or highest level that client can tolerate).	Decreases amount of work needed by you and client to raise him to sitting position.
3. Stand opposite client's hips.	Places your center of gravity nearer client.
4. Turn on a diagonal so you are facing client and far corner of bed.	Reduces twisting of your body, since you are facing direction of movement.
5. Place your feet apart with foot closer to head of bed in front of other foot.	Increases your balance and allows you to transfer your weight as client is brought to sitting position at side of bed.
6. Place arm that is nearer head of bed under client's shoulders, supporting his head and neck.	Maintains alignment of client's head and neck as you bring him to sitting position.
7. Place your other arm over client's thighs. (Fig. 20)	Supports client's hip and prevents him from falling backward during procedure.
8. Move client's lower legs and feet over side of bed.	Decreases friction and resistance during the procedure.
9. Pivot toward your rear leg, allowing client's upper legs to swing downward. (Fig. 21)	Allows gravity to work with you to lower client's legs.

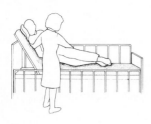

Fig. 20

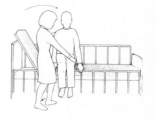

Fig. 21

Steps	Rationale
10. At same time, shift your weight to rear leg and elevate client.	Allows you to transfer your weight in direction of motion.
11. Remain in front of client until he regains balance.	Reduces client's risk of falling.
12. Lower the level of bed until client's feet are touching floor.	Supports client's feet in dorsal flexion and allows client to easily stand at side of bed.
13. Record in nurse's notes client's new position.	Documents that procedure was performed.

Nurse Alert

Clients who have been immobilized or on bedrest are at risk of postural hypotension. The nurse should slowly assist them to a sitting position, being always watchful for the presence of dizziness, light-headedness, or fainting.

Client Teaching

This skill provides the client and family an opportunity to learn the basic mechanics of appropriate body alignment for the sitting position.

Pediatric Considerations

Children usually are easy to move, and the nurse may be able to independently lift a child up in bed.

Geriatric Considerations

Elderly clients with degenerative joint disease (osteoarthritis) are at greater risk than younger clients of shoulder joint dislocation while being assisted up in bed. In addition, because of underlying cardiovascular disease, they may be at increased risk of postural hypotension.

Transferring a Client From Bed to Chair

Transferring a client from bed to chair enables the nurse to change his surroundings as well as his position. If the client is able to tolerate transfer to a wheelchair, the nurse can move him out of his room into other surroundings and increase his opportunities for socialization. For clients who have been on bedrest this is one of the first activities to be resumed.

Potential Nursing Diagnoses

Clients requiring transfer techniques from bed to chair may have one or more of the following nursing diagnoses:

Potential activity intolerance related to limited mobility
Potential impaired skin integrity related to limited mobility
Diversional activity deficit related to limited mobility

Steps	Rationale
1. Assist client to a sitting position on side of bed. Have chair in position with back of chair parallel to head of bed.	Prepares client for move.
2. Place your feet apart.	Ensures better balance.
3. Flex your hips and knees, aligning your knees with client's. (Fig. 22)	Flexion of hips and knees lowers your center of gravity to level of "object" being raised. Aligning your knees with client's allows for stabilization when he stands.
4. Straighten your hips and legs. (Fig. 23)	Uses correct body mechanics to raise client to a standing position.

Steps	Rationale
5. Pivot on foot that is farther from chair, moving client directly in front of chair. (Fig. 24)	Maintains client's support while allowing adequate space for him to move.
6. Instruct client to use armrests on chair for support.	Increases client's stability.
7. Flex your hips and knees while lowering client into chair. (Fig. 25)	Prevents injury to you resulting from poor body mechanics.

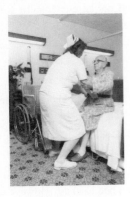

Fig. 22

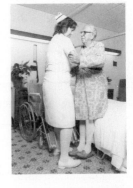

Fig. 23

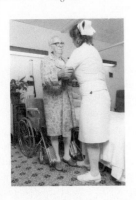

Fig. 24

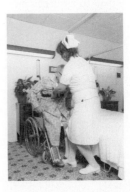

Fig. 25

Steps	Rationale
8. Assess client for proper alignment.	
9. Record in nurse's notes client's safe transfer to chair.	Documents that procedure was performed.

Nurse Alert

Transfer of a client from bed to chair by one nurse requires assistance from the client and should not be attempted if the client is unable to help or to understand the nurse's instructions.

Client Teaching

This is an appropriate time to teach a client and his family the principles of safe transfer technique and body alignment.

Pediatric Considerations

Because children often are easier to move, the nurse may be able to independently lift a child from bed to chair. However, once the child is in the chair, the nurse must reassess his body alignment to ensure proper positioning.

Geriatric Considerations

Physiological changes of aging result in some sensory disturbances that make transferring an elderly client from bed to chair more difficult. First, the client may be increasingly susceptible to postural hypotension, dizziness, and the risk of fainting. Second, changes in his visual and hearing acuity may make it more difficult for him to accurately visualize the chair or understand instructions. Last, decreased balance and changes in the musculoskeletal system increase his risk of falling.

Three-Person Carry

The three-person carry is used to transfer an immobilized or unconscious client from bed to stretcher or bed to bed. This technique is best implemented when all persons doing the lifting are of similar height. Then their centers of gravity will be within the same plane and they can lift as a balanced unit.

Potential Nursing Diagnosis

Clients requiring a three-person carry may have either or both of the following nursing diagnoses:

Impaired physical mobility related to fatigue or decreased level of consciousness

Potential for impaired skin integrity related to limited mobility.

Steps	Rationale
1. Three nurses stand side by side and face client's bed.	Prevents twisting of any nurse's body.
2. Each nurse assumes responsibility for one of three areas: (a) head and shoulders, (b) hips, (c) thighs and ankles.	Distributes client's body weight among lifters.
3. Each assumes wide base of support with foot closer to stretcher in front, knees slightly flexed.	Increases nurses' balance and lowers their center of gravity.
4. Nurses reach under client's head-shoulders,	Distributes client's weight over lifters' forearms.

117

Steps	Rationale
hips, and thighs-ankles, with their fingers secure around side of client's body.	
5. Nurses roll client toward their chests.	Moves workload over lifters' base of support.
6. On count of three, they lift client and hold him against their chests.	Enables nurses to work together and lift safely.
7. On second count of three, they step back and turn toward stretcher, moving as a unit.	Transfers client's weight toward stretcher.
8. Nurses gently lower client onto stretcher by flexing their knees and hips until their elbows are level with edge of stretcher.	Maintains lifters' alignment during transfer.
9. Nurses assess client's body alignment, place safety straps across him, and raise side rails.	Reduces risk of injury to client from poor alignment or falling.
10. Procedure is recorded in nurses' notes.	Documents a safe transfer process.

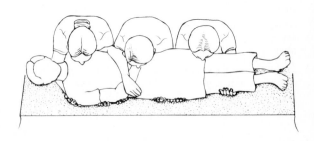

Fig. 26

Nurse Alert

Caution must be used when transferring a client who has undergone surgery or sustained trauma to the spinal cord. If a client with spinal cord injury must be moved, the three-person carry will maintain alignment of the cord during transfer. However, a physician should be in attendance.

Geriatric Considerations

Before transfer, explain to the client specifically how the transfer is to occur. This will orient him as to what he can expect and will reduce his anxiety as well as the chances of injury.

Crutch Walking

Crutches are often needed to increase a client's mobility. The use of crutches may be temporary (such as after ligament damage to the knee) or permanent (as with paralysis of the lower extremities). It is important that crutches be measured for the appropriate length and that clients be taught how to use them correctly.

Potential Nursing Diagnoses

Clients requiring the use of crutches may have one or more of the following nursing diagnoses:

Impaired physical mobility related to trauma to or paralysis of the lower extremities

Potential for injury related to improper use of crutches

Potential for impairment in skin integrity related to improper crutch size

Equipment

Tape measure   Rubber crutch tips
Goniometer   Wooden crutches

Steps	Rationale
1. Wash hands.	Reduces transmission of microorganisms.
2. Measure for crutch length: 3-4 finger widths from axilla to a point 15 cm (6 inches) lateral to client's heel. (Fig. 27)	Ensures that crutches are individualized to client's height.

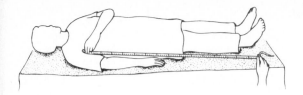

Fig. 27

Steps	Rationale
3. Position crutch handgrips with elbows flexed at 20-25 degree angle. Angle of elbow flexion should be verified by goniometer. (Fig. 28)	Prevents client's body weight from being supported by axillae and consequent nerve damage.
4. Verify that distance between crutch pad and axilla is 3-4 finger widths. (Fig. 29)	Prevents axillary skin breakdown secondary to pressure from crutch pad.
5. Instruct client to assume tripod stance. Tripod stance is formed when crutches are placed 15 cm (6 inches) in front and 15 cm to side of each foot. (Fig. 30)	Improves balance by providing wider base of support. No weight should be borne by axillae.

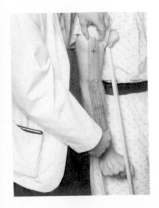

Fig. 28

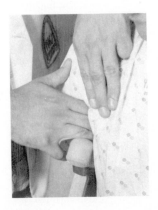

Fig. 29

Steps	Rationale

6. Teach client one of four crutch walking gaits:
 	
    ■ Four-point alternating or four-point gait gives stability to client but requires weight bearing on both legs. Each leg is moved alternately with each crutch so three points of support are on floor at all times. (Fig. 31)
 	
    ■ Three-point alternating or three-point gait requires client to bear all weight on one foot. Weight is borne on uninvolved leg, then on both crutches, and the sequence is repeated. Affected leg does not touch ground during early phase of three-point gait. Gradually client progresses to touchdown and full weight bearing on affected leg. (Fig. 32)
 	
    ■ Two-point gait requires at least partial weight bearing on each foot. Client moves each crutch at same time as opposing leg, so crutch movements are similar to arm motion during normal walking. (Fig. 33)
 	
    ■ Swing-through or swing-to gait is frequently used by paraplegics who wear weight-supporting braces on their legs. With weight on supported
	Allows client to ambulate safely. Specific type of gait chosen depends on client's impairment and physician's order.

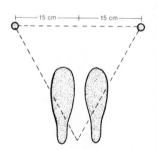

Fig. 30

Steps	Rationale
legs, client places crutches one stride in front and then swings to or through them while they support his weight.	
7. Teach client to ascend and descend on stairs: *Ascend* • Assume a tripod position.	Reduces risk of further damage to musculoskeletal system and risk of falling.

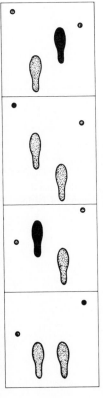

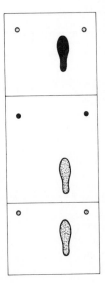

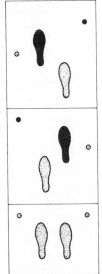

Fig. 31   Fig. 32   Fig. 33

Steps	Rationale
▪ Transfer body weight to crutches. (Fig. 34)	
▪ Advance unaffected leg between crutches and stair.	
▪ Shift weight from crutches to unaffected leg. (Fig. 35)	
▪ Align both crutches on stair. (Fig. 36)	
Descend	
▪ Transfer body weight to unaffected leg. (Fig. 37)	
▪ Place crutches on stair and begin to transfer body weight to crutches, moving affected leg forward. (Fig. 38)	
▪ Align unaffected leg on stair with crutches. (Fig. 39)	
8. Teach client how to sit in chair and how to get up from chair:	Provides safe method of sitting in and getting up from chair. Reduces further damage to client's musculoskeletal system and the risk of falling.
Sitting	
▪ Client positioned at center front of chair with posterior aspects of legs touching chair. (Fig. 40)	
▪ Client holds both crutches in hand opposite affected leg. If both legs are affected, crutches are held in hand on client's stronger side. (Fig. 41)	
▪ Client grasps arm of chair with remaining hand and lowers body into chair. (Fig. 42)	
Getting up	
▪ Perform three steps above in reverse order.	

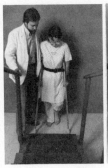

Fig. 34

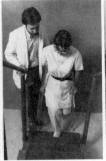

Fig. 35

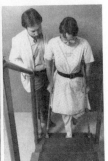

Fig. 36

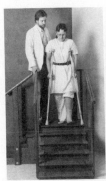

Fig. 37

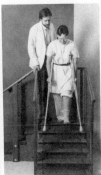

Fig. 38

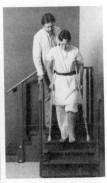

Fig. 39

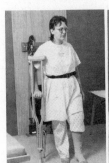

Fig. 40

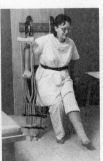

Fig. 41

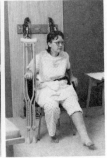

Fig. 42

Steps	Rationale
9. Record in nurse's notes gait and procedures taught and client's ability to perform gaits.	Documents teaching and client's learning.

Nurse Alert

The client with cognitive impairment or who has received analgesics or tranquilizers may be unable to understand instruction or unable to safely ambulate with crutches.

Client Teaching

The nurse should instruct the client that, because of the potential for axillary skin breakdown and nerve damage, he must not lean on his crutches to support his body weight. Rubber crutch tips should be replaced as they wear out, and they should remain dry. Worn or wet crutch tips decrease surface tension and increase the risk of falling. The client should be given a list of medical suppliers in his community so he can obtain repairs as well as new rubber tips, handgrips, and crutch pads. In addition, it is advisable that he have spare crutches and tips on hand.

Geriatric Considerations

The normal visual acuity changes with aging may prevent the client from safely ascending or descending stairs with crutches.

Applying Elastic Stockings

Elastic stockings reduce the risk of thrombus formation. They are available in toe-to-knee and toe-to-midthigh sizes, and they promote venous return by maintaining pressure on the muscles of the lower extremities.

Potential Nursing Diagnoses

Clients requiring elastic stockings may have either or both of the following nursing diagnoses:

Impaired physical mobility related to fatigue or bedrest
Potential activity intolerance related to restricted mobility
Reduced tissue perfusion

Equipment

Talcum powder
Basin and water
Wash cloth and towel
Tape measure
Elastic support stockings in correct size

Steps	Rationale
1. Remove elastic stockings at least twice a day.	Enables you to clean and assess skin and vessels of the legs.
2. After legs have been cleaned, apply a small amount of talcum powder to each leg and foot.	Reduces friction and allows for easier application of stocking.

Steps	Rationale
3. Turn elastic stocking inside out down to foot by placing one hand into sock, holding toe of sock with other hand, and pulling. (Fig. 43)	Allows easier application of stocking.
4. Place client's toe into foot of elastic stocking, making sure that sock is smooth. (Fig. 44)	Wrinkles in sock can impede circulation to lower region of extremity.
5. Slide remaining portion of stocking over client's foot and heel, being sure that his toes are covered. Stocking will now be right side out. (Fig. 45)	If toes remain uncovered, they will become constricted by the elastic and their circulation can be reduced.

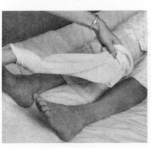

Fig. 43

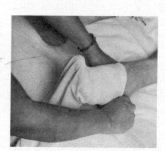

Fig. 44

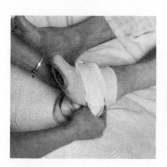

Fig. 45

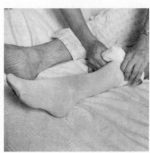

Fig. 46

Steps	Rationale
6. Slide stocking up over client's calf until it completely covers the leg. Be sure that it is smooth and contains no wrinkles. (Fig. 46)	Ridges impede venous return and can counteract overall purpose of elastic stocking.
7. Instruct client not to roll the stockings partially down.	Rolling sock partially down will have a constricting effect and impede venous return.
8. Record in nurses's notes removal and reapplication of elastic stockings, client's skin integrity, and adequacy of circulation to distal extremities.	Documents that procedure was performed.

Nurse Alert

Clients who wear elastic stockings must have the circulation to their distal extremities checked at least every 2 hours. The nurse evaluates the circulation by assessing capillary refill of the great toe. This is done by compressing the nail bed, observing the blanching, and noting the promptness of return to normal color (2 to 3 seconds). If capillary refill is greater than 2 or 3 seconds and the toes are cold, the elastic stockings are impeding circulation and must be removed.

Client Education

This procedure enables the nurse to teach the client good foot care as well as application of elastic stockings for his return home.

Geriatric Considerations

Elastic stockings should not be used, or should be used only with caution, in clients who have chronic peripheral vascular disease, diabetes, or chronic venous leg ulcers.

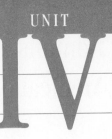

MEDICATIONS

UNIT

IV

Administering an Oral Medication

The oral route is the safest, easiest, and most commonly used method of drug administration. Oral medications are available in various liquid and solid forms, with each type requiring special considerations when given to a client. For example, enteric-coated tablets should never be crushed, syrups should never be followed by liquids, suspensions should be thoroughly shaken before pouring, and sublingual medications should be placed under the client's tongue and allowed to dissolve. Clients who are unable to swallow, who are restricted from taking fluids, who are unconscious, or who have impaired gastrointestinal function cannot be given oral medications.

Potential Nursing Diagnoses

Clients who are taking oral medicines can have any of a variety of nursing diagnoses. Since many clients receive prescribed medications, potential nursing diagnoses may include either or both of the following:

    Knowledge deficit related to drug therapy or to disease condition

    Alteration in health maintenance related to poor drug therapy compliance

Equipment

Medication cards, Kardex, or record form
Medication cart or tray
Disposable medication cups
Glass of water or juice
Drinking straw

Steps	Rationale
1. Gather medication cards or Kardex forms that list all drugs to be given to client at prescribed time.	Cards and forms show which drugs client receives.
2. Check accuracy and completeness of each card or form with physician's written medication order, looking at client's name, drug name and dosage, route of administration, and time for administration.	Physician's order is most reliable resource and the only legal record of drugs client is to receive. NOTE: Check all orders at least every 24 hours.
3. Recopy any card or portion of form that is illegible.	Cards that are soiled or illegible can be source of drug errors.
4. Wash hands.	Removal of microorganisms minimizes their transfer from your hands to medications and equipment.
5. Arrange medication tray and cups in medicine room or move medication cart to position outside client's room.	Organization of equipment saves time and reduces error.
6. Unlock medicine drawer or cart.	Medications are safeguarded when locked in cabinet or cart.
7. Prepare medications for one client at a time. Keep medication tickets or forms for each client together.	Prevents preparation errors.
8. Select correct drug from stock or unit dose drawer and compare with medication card or form.	Reading label against transcribed order reduces error.
9. Calculate correct dosage.	Calculation will be more accurate when information from drug labels is at hand.

Steps	Rationale
10. If administering tablets or capsules from bottle, pour required number into bottle cap and transfer to medication cup. *Do not touch medicines with your fingers.* Extra tablets or capsules may be returned to bottle.	Aseptic technique maintains cleanliness of drugs.
11. Transfer unit-dose–packaged tablets or capsules to a medication cup. (Do not remove wrapper.) All tablets or capsules given to client at same time may be placed in one cup except for those requiring preadministration assessments (such as pulse rate and blood pressure).	Keeping medications that require preadministration assessments separate from others will make it easier to withhold those drugs if necessary.
12. To pour liquids, remove bottle cap and place it upside down.	Prevents contamination.
13. Hold bottle with label against palm of hand while pouring.	Spilled liquid will not soil or fade label.
14. Hold medication cup at eye level and fill to desired mark. (Scale should be even with fluid at bottom of meniscus.) (Fig. 47)	Ensures accuracy of measurement.

Fig. 47

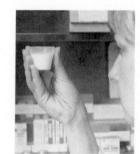

Steps	Rationale
15. Discard excess liquid into sink. Wipe lip of bottle with paper towel.	Prevents contamination of bottle's contents and keeps bottle cap from sticking.
16. When preparing narcotic, check narcotic record for previous drug count, remove required volume of drug, record necessary information on form, and sign form.	Controlled substance laws require careful monitoring of dispensed narcotics.
17. Compare medication card or form with prepared drug and container.	Reading label a second time reduces error.
18. Return stock containers or unused unit-dose medications to shelf or drawer and read labels third time.	Reduces administration error.
19. Place medications and cards together on tray or cart.	Drugs are labeled at all times for identification.
20. Do not leave drugs unattended.	You are responsible for safekeeping of drugs.
21. Take medications to client at correct time.	Medications are administered within period of 30 minutes before or 30 minutes after prescribed time to ensure intended therapeutic effect.
22. Identify client by comparing name on card or form with name on client's identification band. Ask client to state his name.	Identification bands are made at time of client's admission and are most reliable source of identification. Replace any missing ID bands.
23. Perform any necessary preadministration assessment.	Determines whether medications should be given at that time.
24. Explain purpose of medication and its action to client.	Client's understanding of purpose of medication will improve compliance with drug therapy.

Steps	Rationale
25. Assist client to sitting or side-lying position.	This prevents aspiration during swallowing.
26. Administer drugs properly. Offer client choice of water or juice with drugs to be swallowed. Client may wish to hold solid medications in hand or cup before placing in mouth.	Choice of therapy promotes client comfort. Client can become familiar with medications by seeing each drug and then will be able to recognize correct drugs.
27. If client is unable to hold medications, place medication up to his lips and gently introduce drugs into his mouth.	Prevents contamination of medications.
28. If tablet or capsule falls to floor, discard it and repeat preparation.	Prevents contamination.
29. Stay with client until he has completely swallowed each medication. If uncertain whether medication was swallowed, ask client to open his mouth.	You are responsible for ensuring that client receives ordered dose. If left unattended, client may not take dose or may save drugs, causing risk to his health.
30. Wash your hands.	Reduces spread of microorganisms.
31. Record each drug administered on medication record.	Prompt documentation prevents errors such as repeated doses.
32. Return medication cards to appropriate file for next administration time.	Cards are used as reference for when next dose is due. Loss of card may lead to administration error.
33. Discard used supplies, replenish stock (e.g., cups and straws), and clean work area.	Clean working space assists other staff in completing duties efficiently.

Steps	Rationale
34. Return within 30 minutes to evaluate client's response to medications.	By monitoring client's response, you will assess drug's therapeutic benefit and be able to detect onset of side effects or allergic reactions.

Nurse Alert

If the client begins coughing during drug administration, stop immediately. Aspiration of medication or fluid can easily occur.

Client Teaching

Clients may require extensive instruction on how to take prescribed medications correctly. They should understand the purpose of each medication, its action and potential side effects, and the correct time and frequency of its administration. They should particularly understand what can happen if they arbitrarily omit a dose or cease taking the medication entirely. They should also know whether to take medications before or after meals.

When attempting to establish medication schedules, consider the client's home environment and daily routines. Clients with visual alterations may be unable to read printed labels and thus require large-print instructions. Include family members in the teaching in case a client becomes too ill to self-administer drugs reliably.

Pediatric Considerations

Children unable to swallow or chew solid medications should be given only liquid preparations. Generally it is safe to administer solid drug forms to children 5 years or older. Pediatric preparations are usually colorful and pleasant tasting. However, a child may enjoy a "chaser" of juice, carbonated soft drink, or frozen juice bar. A bad-tasting drug can be mixed in jam, syrup, or honey. Oral medications are most easily administered to infants by spoon, plastic cup or dropper, or small plastic syringe.

Geriatric Considerations

Elderly clients often have multiple medications prescribed. It can be quite helpful to set specific time schedules convenient with their daily routines so they do not forget to take a dose. Many elderly clients have mobility and sensory limitations that prohibit safe drug preparation and administration, and family member or friend should be available for assistance.

Preparing an Injectable Medication From an Ampule

An ampule is a clear glass container with a constricted neck. It contains a single dose of a medication in liquid form. The nurse must snap off the ampule's neck to gain access to the medication. When withdrawing the medication, the nurse uses aseptic technique (by preventing the needle from touching the ampule's outer surface). Fluid can be aspirated easily into the syringe by simply drawing back on the syringe plunger.

Potential Nursing Diagnoses

This procedure may be performed by nurses caring for clients with a variety of nursing diagnoses.

Equipment

Syringe and needle of desired size
Ampule of prescribed medication
Alcohol swab or 2 × 2 gauze pad
Metal file (optional)
Extra sterile needle.

Steps	Rationale
1. Wash hands.	Reduces transmission of microorganisms.
2. Tap top of ampule lightly and quickly with a finger. (Fig. 48)	Dislodges any fluid that collects above neck. All solution moves into lower chamber.

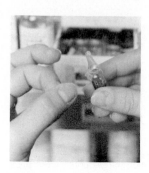

Fig. 48

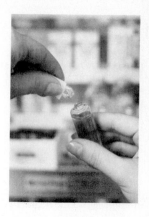

Fig. 49

Steps	Rationale
3. Place small gauze pad or dry alcohol swab around neck of ampule.	Protects fingers from trauma as glass is broken.
4. Snap neck of ampule away from your hands. (If neck does not break, use a file to score one side of it.) (Fig. 49).	Prevents shattering glass toward your fingers or face.
5. Hold ampule either inverted or right side up. Insert needle into center of ampule opening. Do not allow needle tip or shaft to touch rim of ampule. NOTE: Ampule may be held inverted as long as needle tip or shaft does not touch its rim.	Broken rim of ampule is considered contaminated.
6. Aspirate medication into syringe by pulling back on plunger.	Withdrawal of plunger creates a negative pressure within barrel that pulls fluid into syringe.

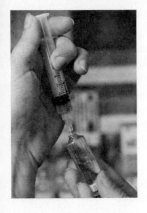

Fig. 50

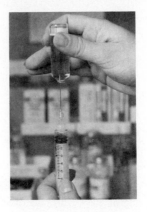

Fig. 51

Steps	Rationale
7. Keep needle tip below surface of liquid. If holding ampule upright, tip it to bring all fluid within reach of needle. (Fig. 50)	Prevents aspiration of air bubbles.
8. If air bubbles are aspirated, do not expel air into ampule.	Air pressure will force fluid out of ampule, and medication will be lost.
9. To expel excess air bubbles, remove needle from ampule. Hold syringe with needle pointing up. Draw back slightly on plunger and push it upward to eject air. *Do not eject fluid.* (Fig. 51)	Withdrawing plunger too far will pull it from barrel. Holding syringe vertically allows fluid to settle in bottom of barrel. Pulling back on plunger allows fluid within needle to enter barrel.
10. After withdrawing required fluid volume, remove needle from ampule. Hold syringe and needle upright and tap syringe barrel to dislodge air bubbles. Eject air as described in Step 9.	Air within barrel displaces medication and causes dosage errors.

Steps	Rationale
11. Change sterile needle.	Prevents tracking of medication into tissues. Original needle's outer surface is coated with medication.
12. Cover needle with its sheath or cap.	Prevents contamination of needle and prevents needle sticks.

Nurse Alert

Use caution when snapping off the neck of an ampule. Shattering of glass can injure your fingers.

Preparing an Injectable Medication From a Vial

A vial is a single- or multiple-dose glass container with a rubber seal at the top. It can contain either a liquid or a dry drug preparation. Drugs that are unstable in solution are packaged in dry form. The vial label specifies the type of solvent used to dissolve the drug and the amount needed to prepare a desired drug concentration.

Unlike the ampule, the vial is a closed system. Air must first be injected into the vial for fluid to be easily withdrawn. Failure to inject air when withdrawing solution creates a vacuum within the vial that makes withdrawal difficult.

Potential Nursing Diagnoses

The procedure of preparing an injectable medication from a vial may be performed by nurses caring for clients with a variety of nursing diagnoses.

Equipment

Syringe and needle of desired size
Alcohol swab
Vial with prescribed medication
Extra sterile needle
Label

Steps	Rationale
1. Wash hands.	Reduces transmission of microorganisms.
2. Remove metal cap to expose rubber seal.	Vial comes packaged with cap to prevent contamination of seal.
3. With alcohol swab, wipe off surface of rubber seal.	Removes dust or grease but does not sterilize surface.
4. Remove needle cap. Pull back on plunger to draw air into syringe equivalent to volume of medication to be aspirated. (Fig. 52)	To prevent buildup of negative pressure when aspirating medication, you must first inject air into vial.
5. Insert tip of needle, with bevel pointing up, through center of rubber seal. Apply pressure to needle point during insertion. (Fig. 53)	Center of seal is thinner and easier to penetrate. Keeping bevel up and using firm pressure prevent cutting rubber core from seal.
6. Inject air into vial, holding on to plunger.	Air must be injected first before aspirating fluid. Plunger may be forced backward by air pressure within vial.

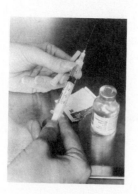

Fig. 52

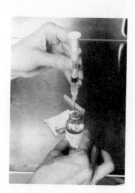

Fig. 53

Steps	Rationale
7. Invert vial while keeping firm hold on syringe and plunger. Hold vial between thumb and middle finger of nondominant hand. Grasp end of barrel and plunger with thumb and forefinger of dominant hand.	Inverting vial allows fluid to settle in lower half of container. Position of hands prevents movement of plunger and permits easy manipulation of syringe.
8. Keep tip of needle below fluid level.	Prevents aspiration of air.
9. Allow air pressure to gradually fill syringe with medication. Pull back slightly on plunger if necessary. (Fig. 54)	Positive pressure within vial forces fluid into syringe.
10. Tap side of barrel carefully to dislodge any air bubbles. Eject any air remaining at top of syringe into vial.	Forcefully striking barrel while needle is inserted in vial may bend needle. Accumulation of air displaces medication and causes dosage errors.
11. To expel excess air bubbles, remove needle from	Withdrawing plunger too far will pull it from barrel. Hold-

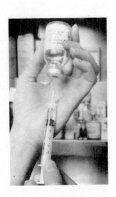

Fig. 54

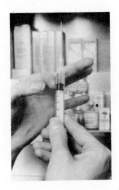

Fig. 55

Steps	Rationale
vial by pulling back on barrel. Hold syringe with needle pointing up and tap it to dislodge bubbles. Draw back slightly on plunger and push plunger upward to eject air. *Do not eject fluid.* (Fig. 55)	ing syringe vertically allows fluid to settle in bottom of barrel. Pulling back on plunger allows fluid within needle to enter barrel.
12. Change sterile needle.	Pushing needle through rubber stopper may dull needle tip.
13. Cover needle with its sheath or cap.	Prevents contamination of the needle.
14. Label vial if any medication remains. Note amount of solution and concentration of drug.	Ensures accurate drug administration when successive doses are given.

Nurse Alert

Be sure that air pressure does not force the plunger out of the syringe barrel. This causes contamination of the syringe.

Administering Subcutaneous and Intramuscular Injections

The administration of an injection is an invasive procedure involving deposition of medication through a sterile needle inserted into body tissues. Aseptic technique must be maintained since a client is at risk of infection once the needle penetrates the skin. The characteristics of tissues influence the rate of drug absorption and onset of drug action. Thus, before injecting a drug the nurse should know the volume of medication to administer, the characteristics of the drug, and the location of anatomical structures underlying injection sites.

For subcutaneous injections, medication is deposited into the loose connective tissue under the dermis. Since the subcutaneous tissue is not richly supplied with blood vessels, drug absorption is somewhat slower than with intramuscular injections. Subcutaneous tissues contain pain receptors so only small doses of water-soluble nonirritating medications should be given by this route.

The intramuscular route provides faster drug absorption because of a muscle's vascularity. The danger of tissue damage is less when medications enter deep muscle. Muscles also are less sensitive to irritating and viscous drugs. However, there is a risk of inadvertently injecting into a blood vessel if the nurse is not careful.

Potential Nursing Diagnoses

Clients receiving injections may have any of a number of nursing diagnoses. When a client receives an injection, he is at risk of the following:

Potential for injury related to needle trauma or infection

Alteration in comfort related to nerve trauma

Equipment

Syringe (size varies according to volume of drug to be administered)

Needle (size varies according to type of tissue and size of client; intramuscular—20 to 23 gauge and ⅝ to 1½ inches in length; subcutaneous—25 to 27 gauge and ½ to ⅞ inch in length)

Antiseptic swab, e.g., alcohol

Medication ampule or vial

Medication card or form

Steps	Rationale
1. Wash hands.	Reduces transmission of microorganisms.
2. Assemble equipment and check medication order for route, dose, and time.	Ensures accuracy of order.
3. Prepare medication from ampule or vial as described in Skills 4-2 and 4-3.	Ensures that medication is sterile.
4. Check client's identification band and ask client's name.	Ensures that right client receives right drug.
5. Explain procedure to client and proceed in calm manner.	Helps client anticipate nurse's actions.
6. Select appropriate injection site. Palpate site for edema, masses, or tenderness. Avoid areas of scarring, bruising, abrasion, or infection. (Fig. 56)	Injection sites should be free of lesions that might interfere with drug absorption. Sufficient muscle mass is needed to ensure accurate intramuscular injection into proper tissue.

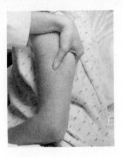

Fig. 56

Steps	Rationale
• When administering heparin subcutaneously, use abdominal injection sites.	NOTE: Anticoagulants may cause local bleeding and bruising when injected into areas such as arms and legs, which are involved in muscular activity.
• For intramuscular injection, palpate muscles to determine their firmness and size.	
7. In cases of repeated daily insulin injections, do not use same injection site. Rotate within a single anatomical region and then change anatomical site. Do not reuse same site within 3-week period.	Rotation of site prevents subcutaneous scarring and lipodystrophy, which can interfere with drug absorption.
8. Assist client to comfortable position depending on site chosen:	
Subcutaneous injection Arm—client sitting or standing Abdomen—client sitting or supine Leg—client sitting in bed or chair	Provides easy access to site with client in relaxed position.

Steps	Rationale
Intramuscular injection Thigh (vastus lateralis)—client lying supine with knee slightly flexed Ventrogluteal—client on side, back, or abdomen with knee and hip on side to be injected flexed Dorsogluteal—client prone with feet turned inward or on side with upper knee and hip flexed and placed in front of lower leg Shoulder (deltoid)—client sitting or lying flat with lower arm flexed but relaxed across abdomen or lap	Helping client assume position that reduces strain on muscle will minimize discomfort of injection.
9. Ask client to relax his arm or leg, whichever site is chosen. Talk with him about subject of interest.	Minimizes discomfort during injection. Distraction helps reduce anxiety.
10. Relocate site using anatomical landmarks.	Accurate injection requires insertion in correct anatomical site to avoid injuring underlying nerves, bones, or blood vessels.
11. Clean the site with antiseptic swab. Apply swab at center of site and rotate outward in circular direction for about 5 cm (2 inches). (Fig. 57)	Mechanical action of swab removes secretions containing microorganisms.
12. Hold swab between third and fourth fingers of your nondominant hand.	Swab will remain readily accessible when time to withdraw needle.
13. Remove needle cap from syringe by pulling cap straight off.	Prevents needle from touching sides of cap and becoming contaminated.

Steps	Rationale
14. Hold syringe between thumb and forefinger of your dominant hand as though it were a dart. (Most nurses hold syringe palm up for subcutaneous injections and palm down for intramuscular injections because of different angles of insertion.) (Fig. 58)	Quick smooth injection requires proper manipulation of syringe parts.
15. Inject syringe: *Subcutaneous*	
▪ For average-sized client, with your non-dominant hand either spread skin tightly across injection site or pinch skin.	Needle penetrates tight skin more easily than loose skin. Pinching skin elevates subcutaneous tissue.
▪ Inject needle quickly and firmly at a 45-degree angle. (Then release skin if pinched)	Quick firm insertion minimizes client anxiety and discomfort.

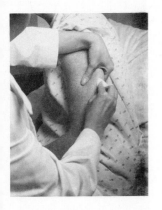

Fig. 57

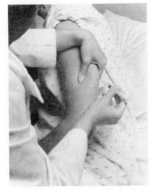

Fig. 58

Steps	Rationale
▪ For obese client, pinch skin at site and inject needle below tissue fold.	Obese clients have fatty layer of tissue above subcutaneous tissue.
Intramuscular	
▪ Position nondominant hand at proper anatomical landmarks and spread skin tightly. Inject needle quickly at a 90-degree angle.	Speeds insertion and reduces discomfort.
▪ If muscle mass is small, grasp body of muscle and inject medication.	Ensures that medication reaches muscle tissue.
▪ If giving irritating preparation, use Z-track method. Pull overlying skin and subcutaneous tissues 2.5-3.5 cm (1-1½ inches) laterally to side. Hold skin back and inject needle quickly.	Creates zig-zag path through tissues that seals needle track to avoid tracking medication through sensitive subcutaneous tissues.
16. Once needle enters site, with your nondominant hand grasp lower end of syringe barrel. Move your dominant hand to end of plunger. Avoid movement of syringe. (Fig. 59)	Properly performed injection requires smooth manipulation of syringe parts. Movement of syringe may displace needle and cause discomfort.
▪ If giving Z track, keep tight hold of skin with nondominant hand. Use dominant hand to carefully move toward plunger.	Skin must remain pulled until drug injected.
17. Slowly pull back on plunger to aspirate medication. If blood appears in syringe, withdraw nee-	Aspiration of blood into syringe indicates intravenous placement of needle. Subcutaneous and intramuscular medi-

Steps	Rationale
dle, dispose of syringe, and repeat medication preparation. If no blood appears, inject medication slowly. NOTE: Some agencies recommend not aspirating subcutaneous heparin injections.	cations are not for intravenous use. Slow injection reduces pain and tissue trauma. NOTE: Heparin is an anticoagulant that is typically given in small subcutaneous doses. The drug may cause bruising when aspirated. The drug is not harmful if given intravenously.
18. Withdraw needle quickly while placing antiseptic swab just above injection site. (Fig. 60) ■ When using Z-track, keep needle inserted after injecting drug for 10 sec. Then release skin after withdrawing needle.	Support of tissues around the injection site minimizes discomfort during needle withdrawal. Allows medication to disperse evenly. Tissue planes slide across one another to create zig-zag path that seals medication into muscle tissues.
19. Massage site lightly.	Massage stimulates circulation and thus improves drug distribution and absorption.

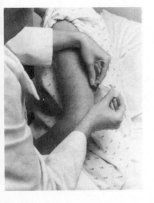

Fig. 59

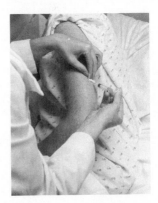

Fig. 60

Steps	Rationale
20. Assist client to a comfortable position.	Gives client sense of well-being.
21. Discard needle and syringe into appropriately labeled receptacles.	Prevents injury to client and hospital personnel. Capping needle can cause needle stick.
22. Wash hands.	Controls spread of infection.
23. Chart medication in medication sheet or nurse's notes.	Prevents future drug errors.
24. Return to evaluate client's response to medication within 15-30 minutes.	Parenteral drugs are absorbed and act more quickly than oral medications. Your observations determine efficacy of drug action.

Nurse Alert

The needle of the syringe must remain sterile before insertion. During aspiration if blood appears in the syringe, immediately withdraw and start over. Document and report any sudden localized pain or burning at the injection site, which may indicate nerve injury.

Client Teaching

The insulin-dependent client may have to learn how to self-administer injections if family members are not available. It may be necessary to teach him aseptic principles, the basic pharmacology of insulin, the selection and rotation of injection sites, and injection techniques.

Pediatric Considerations

When it is essential to deliver a prescribed volume of solution to a child, draw up 0.2 ml of air into the syringe after preparing the drug dose. Air acts as dead space to clear the needle bore of medication. Give parents the option of helping to restrain their child during an injection. Some parents do not wish to be looked upon as the ones causing the child discomfort. It may help to keep the needle out of the child's line of vision to minimize anxiety. Never surprise a child. Be sure that he knows he is to receive an injection. The vastus lateralis is the preferred injection site for children. After the injection, provide comfort to the child.

Geriatric Considerations

The elderly client's muscle mass may be reduced. It is therefore important to choose a proper-sized needle. Remember also that the elderly client may be unable to tolerate more than 2 ml of an intramuscular injection.

Adding Medication to an Intravenous Fluid Container

The safest method for administering intravenous medications is to add the drugs to large-volume fluid containers (usually with dextrose and water solution or normal saline). Then the medication infuses slowly, the risk of side effects is minimized, and therapeutic blood levels are maintained. Drugs added to intravenous fluid containers include electrolytes, vitamins, and minerals. The primary risk involved with infusing drugs by this method is fluid overload.

Potential Nursing Diagnoses

Nursing diagnoses of which the nurse should be aware when caring for clients who are receiving medications through large-volume intravenous infusion containers include the following:

Potential for injury related to administration of IV medications

Potential for fluid volume excess related to IV infusion

Equipment

Prepared medication in syringe

Intravenous fluid container (bag or bottle, 500 or 1000 ml volume)

Alcohol or antiseptic swab

Label to attach to IV bag or bottle

Steps	Rationale
Adding Medication to New Container	
1. Wash hands.	Reduces transmission of microorganisms.
2. Explain procedure to client.	Reduces client anxiety.
3. Check client's identification by reading his ID band and asking his name.	Ensures that right client gets prescribed medication.
BAG	
4. Locate medication injection port on intravenous fluid bag.	The medication injection port is self-sealing to prevent introduction of microorganisms after repeated use.
5. Wipe off port with alcohol or antiseptic swab.	Reduces risk of introducing microorganisms into bag during needle insertion.
6. Carefully insert needle of syringe through center of injection port and depress plunger. (Fig. 61)	Injection of needle into sides of port may produce leak and lead to contamination of fluid.
7. Withdraw syringe and mix solution by holding the bag and turning it gently from end to end.	Allows medication to be distributed evenly throughout bag.

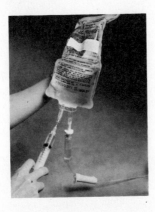

Fig. 61

Steps	Rationale
8. Hang bag and check infusion rate	Prevents rapid infusion of fluid.
9. Complete medication label and stick it upside down on bag.	Label can be easily read during infusion. It alerts nurses to drug in bag.

BOTTLE

4. Remove metal or plastic cap and rubber disk. Place cap upside down on counter top.	Cap seals bottle to maintain its sterility. Inside of cap may remain sterile for reuse.
5. Locate medication injection site on bottle's rubber stopper. Site is usually marked by "X" or circle. Air vent and main tubing port are not injection sites.	Accidental injection through main tubing port or air vent can alter pressure within bottle and cause fluid leaks through air vent.
6. Perform Steps 5 through 9 above.	

Adding Medication to Existing Container
VENTED BOTTLE OR PLASTIC BAG

1. Check volume of solution remaining in container.	Proper volume is needed to adequately dilute medication.
2. Close off IV infusion clamp.	Prevents medication from directly entering client's circulation during injection.
3. Wipe off medication port with alcohol or antiseptic swab.	Mechanically removes microorganisms that could enter container during needle insertion.
4. Insert syringe needle through port and inject medication. (Fig. 62)	Injection port is self-sealing and prevents fluid leaks.
5. Lower container from IV pole and gently mix.	Ensures that medication is evenly distributed throughout bag.
6. Rehang and regulate infusion to desired rate.	Prevents rapid infusion of fluid.
7. Label container with name and dosage of medication.	Alerts other nurses to drug in bag.

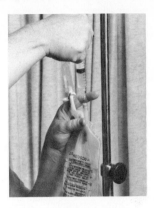

Fig. 62

Nurse Alert

Be aware of the signs and symptoms of fluid overload in case you discover that an excess amount of fluid has infused too quickly. These include tachycardia, bounding pulse, jugular venous distention, and shortness of breath.

Client Teaching

To prevent unnecessary anxiety, the nurse should explain to the client that medications are being added to an existing IV line.

Pediatric Considerations

Infants and children are very susceptible to fluid overload, so infusions must be frequently monitored.

Geriatric Considerations

Although the conditions of renal and heart failure are not limited to the elderly population, it is especially important to consider these clients' risk for fluid overload.

Administering a Medication by Intravenous Bolus

Administration of concentrated medications directly into a vein by the bolus technique is the most dangerous method for drug administration. Drugs act rapidly since they directly enter the client's circulation. Serious side effects can occur within seconds. Therefore it is imperative that the nurse time the administrations carefully to prevent too rapid an infusion. Drugs may be given intravenously through a heparin lock or an existing intravenous infusion line. Intravenous drugs are often given by bolus in emergency situations when rapid actions are desired. The technique is also used to avoid mixing medications that are incompatible.

Potential Nursing Diagnoses

Nursing diagnoses of which to be aware when administering medications by intravenous bolus include the following:

Potential for injury related to administration of IV bolus

Alteration in comfort related to infiltration or needle displacement (indicates need to change IV site before drug administration)

Equipment

Heparin lock

Prepared medication in syringe with small-gauge (25 or 26) needle

Syringe containing 1 ml of 1:1000 heparin solution

Alcohol or antiseptic swab

Watch with second hand or digital readout

Intravenous infusion line
Prepared medication in syringe with small-gauge (25 or 26)
  needle
Alcohol or antiseptic swab
Intravenous line tubing with injection port
Watch with second hand or digital readout

Steps	Rationale
1. Wash hands.	Reduces transmission of infection.
2. Explain procedure to client.	Reduces any anxiety client may have.
3. Check client's identification by reading identification band and asking client's name.	Ensures that right client receives right medication.

Heparin Lock

4. Clean hep lock's rubber diaphragm with antiseptic swab.	Prevents introduction of microorganisms during needle insertion.
5. Insert 25-gauge needle of syringe containing prepared drug through center of diaphragm. (Fig. 63)	Prevents damage to diaphragm and subsequent leakage.
6. Inject medication bolus slowly over several minutes. (Each medication has recommended rate for bolus administration. Check package directions.) Use watch to time administration.	Rapid injection could prove fatal to client.

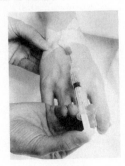

Fig. 63

Steps	Rationale
7. After administering bolus, withdraw syringe. Insert 25-gauge needle of syringe containing diluted heparin (heparin flush) solution. Inject this.	Maintains patency of needle by inhibiting clot formation. Dilution of heparin solution prevents systemic anticoagulation of client.
8. Observe client closely for any adverse reactions.	IV medications act rapidly.
9. Dispose of syringe and needle in proper receptacle.	Prevents accidental injury from needle sticks.
10. Wash hands.	Reduces transmission of microorganisms
11. Record in medication record drug administered.	Prompt documentation prevents drug errors.

Intravenous Infusion Line

1. Determine if IV fluids are infusing at proper rate.	Infusion must be at prescribed rate for therapeutic effect.
2. Select injection port of tubing closest to needle insertion site. (Fig. 64)	Allows for easier fluid aspiration to obtain blood return.

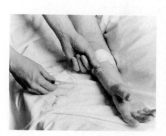
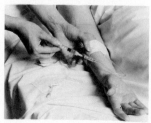

Fig. 64   Fig. 65

Steps	Rationale
3. Clean off injection port with antiseptic swab.	Prevents introduction of microorganisms during needle insertion.
4. Insert small-gauge needle containing prepared drug through center of port. (Fig. 65)	Prevents damage to port's diaphragm and subsequent leakage.
5. Occlude intravenous line by pinching tubing just above injection port. Pull back gently on syringe's plunger to aspirate for blood return. (Fig. 66)	Ensures that medication is being delivered into bloodstream.
6. After noting blood return, release tubing and inject medication slowly over several minutes. (Read directions on drug package.) Use a watch to time administration. (Fig. 67)	Allows slow infusion of fluids. Rapid injection could prove fatal to client.
7. After injecting medication, withdraw syringe and recheck infusion rate.	Injection of bolus may alter rate of fluid infusion. Rapid infusion can cause circulatory overload.

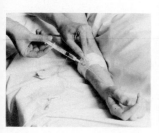

Fig. 66

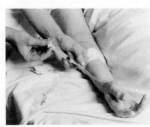

Fig. 67

Steps	Rationale
8. Dispose of needle and syringe in proper receptacles.	Prevents accidental needle sticks and reduces transfer of infection.
9. Observe client closely for adverse reactions.	IV bolus medications act rapidly.
10. Wash your hands.	Reduces transfer of microorganisms.
11. Record in medication record drug administered.	Prompt documentation prevents drug errors.

Nurse Alert

Watch the IV site during drug injection. The sudden development of swelling indicates infiltration. Then it is imperative to stop the injection. It is also imperative to know each drug's side effects and to watch the client for any reaction.

Client Teaching

The nurse may wish to inform a client on the anticipated effects of a medication. For example, an analgesic can bring rapid pain relief and it may help to encourage the client that his discomfort will soon be lessened.

Pediatric Considerations

Remember, an infant's veins are small and fragile. Rapid injection can cause infiltration.

Geriatric Considerations

An elderly client's veins are generally more fragile than a younger client's, and infiltration may occur if fluid is forced too rapidly.

Administering an Intravenous Medication by "Piggyback" or Small-Volume Container

With administration of intravenous medications through piggyback or small-volume containers, there is less risk of causing sudden drug side effects. Medications infuse slowly over several minutes. This technique also prevents the need to infuse large volumes of fluid for clients who have fluid restrictions. The piggyback technique also avoids the need to mix drugs with others that may be incompatible. It is important that the existing intravenous line be infusing properly to ensure proper drug distribution.

Potential Nursing Diagnoses

Nursing diagnoses of which to be aware when administering medications by piggyback or small-volume containers include the following:

Pain at IV insertion site related to phlebitis or infiltration

Potential for injury related to administration of IV medications

Potential for injury related to infection

Equipment

Infusion through adjacent line

Medication prepared in a 50 or 100 ml infusion bag with IV infusion tubing set

165

Main IV infusion line
Needle (21 or 23 gauge)
Alcohol or antiseptic swab
Infusion through Volutrol
Volutrol (plastic graduated container that is part of a main IV line and hangs between main IV bag or bottle and infusion tubing)
Syringe with prepared medication
Alcohol or antiseptic swab

Steps	Rationale
1. Review physician's orders for name of drug and dosage.	Ensures safe and accurate drug administration.
2. Wash hands.	Reduces transmission of microorganisms.
3. Check client's identification band and ask client's name.	Ensures that right client receives right medication.

Infusion Through Adjacent Line

1. Prepare secondary infusion line, being sure tubing is completely filled with medication-fluid mixture.	Prevents introduction of air into primary IV line.
2. Check infusion rate of main IV line.	Checking infusion rate determines patency of system. Any obstruction to flow will interfere with medication delivery.
3. Hang secondary fluid bag at or above level of main fluid bag. (Fig. 68)	Height of fluid bag regulates rate of fluid flow to client.
4. Connect needle to the end of secondary line tubing. Clean injection port to main IV line with an antiseptic swab.	Prevents introduction of microorganisms during needle insertion.
5. Insert needle of secondary line through injection port of main IV line. Regulate	Provides direct route for slow intermittent medication infusion. For optimal therapeutic

Steps	Rationale
flow rate of medication solution (usually 30 to 60 min). (Fig. 69)	effect, drug should infuse within 30-60 minutes.
6. Observe client for signs of adverse reactions.	IV medications act rapidly.
7. After medication has infused, turn off flow regulator on secondary IV line. Leave needle, tubing, and secondary bag hanging for future drug administration.	Secondary line is route for microorganisms to enter main line. Repeated changes of tubing or needle increase risk of infection transmission.
8. Record in medication record drug administered.	Prompt documentation prevents drug errors.

Infusion Through Volutrol

1. Check infusion rate of IV line.	Determines patency of system. Obstruction to flow interferes with medication delivery.
2. Fill Volutrol with desired amount of fluid (50-100 ml) by opening clamp between Volutrol and main IV bag. (Fig. 70)	Small volume of fluid dilutes IV medication and reduces risk of rapid dose infusion.

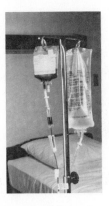

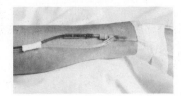

Fig. 68   Fig. 69

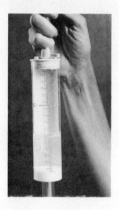

Fig. 70

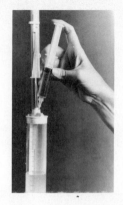

Fig. 71

Steps	Rationale
3. Clean off injection port on top of Volutrol.	Prevents introduction of microorganisms during needle insertion.
4. Insert syringe needle into port and inject medication. (Fig. 71) Gently rotate Volutrol between your hands.	Mixes medication within Volutrol to ensure equal distribution.
5. Recheck IV infusion rate (medication should infuse in 30 to 60 min).	For optimal therapeutic effect drug should infuse within 30 to 60 minutes.
6. Observe client for signs of adverse reactions.	IV medications act rapidly.
7. Record drug administered in medication record.	Prompt documentation prevents drug errors.
8. After medication has infused, refill Volutrol with intravenous solution and monitor flow rate as ordered.	Keeps IV line patent.

Nurse Alert

Know the potential side effects of a medication. Drugs can act rapidly.

Client Teaching

Explain the purpose and actions of a medication to the client.

Pediatric Considerations

Pediatric doses are small. Be sure that the child receives the medication in the Volutrol as well as that in the tubing. An infant or child may not receive as much infusion as an adult because of the risk of fluid overload.

Geriatric Considerations

The veins of an elderly client are fragile. Infiltration at the IV site can develop easily. Observe the site periodically during any intermittent drug infusion.

Topical Skin Applications

A variety of pharmacological preparations can be applied to the client's skin for several purposes: maintaining hydration of skin layers, protecting skin surfaces, reducing local skin irritation, creating local anesthesia, treating sites of infection. Each type of preparation must be applied in a specific way to ensure the medication's proper penetration and absorption. As a client's skin condition changes, a new form of preparation may be ordered by the physician.

The nurse should recognize that a client with alterations of skin integrity may be acutely conscious of his body image changes. Applying topical medications when possible with ungloved hands will convey a feeling of acceptance. The nurse should never show an aversion to inspecting a client's skin's condition or to providing the necessary hygienic care.

Potential Nursing Diagnoses

Clients requiring administration of topical skin applications may have any of the following nursing diagnoses:

Actual impairment of skin integrity related to specific skin alteration

Knowledge deficit regarding purpose and use of topical agents

Alteration in comfort related to skin irritation

Alteration in body image related to skin disorder

Equipment

Ordered topical agent (e.g., cream, ointment, lotion, aerosol, spray, powder)

Medication ticket or form

Small sterile gauze dressings
Disposable or sterile gloves (optional)
Cotton-tipped applicator or tongue blade
Basin with warm water, washcloth, towel, and nondrying
  soap
Gauze dressings, plastic wrap, tape

Steps	Rationale
1. Review physician's order for name of drug, strength, time of administration, and site of application.	Ensures that drug will be administered safely and accurately.
2. Wash hands.	Reduces transmission of infection.
3. Arrange supplies at client's bedside.	Topical agents are not usually premeasured in medication room.
4. Close room curtain or door.	Provides for client privacy.
5. Check client's identification by reading ID bracelet and asking client's name.	Ensures that right client receives prescribed medication.
6. Position client comfortably. Remove gown or bed linen, keeping unaffected areas draped.	Provides for easy access to area being treated. Promotes client comfort.
7. Inspect condition of client's skin thoroughly. Wash any affected area, removing all debris and crustations. (Use mild nondrying soap.)	Provides baseline to determine change in skin's condition following therapy. Skin should be clean for a proper assessment. Removal of debris enhances penetration of topical drug through skin. Cleaning removes microorganisms resident in debris.
8. Pat skin dry or allow area to air dry.	Excess moisture can interfere with even application of topical agent.

Steps	Rationale
9. If skin is excessively dry and flaking, apply topical agent while still damp.	Retains moisture within skin layers.
10. Don gloves if indicated.	Sterile gloves are used when applying agents to open non-infected skin lesions. Disposable gloves prevent cross-contamination of infected or contagious lesions.
11. Apply topical agent: *Cream, ointment, and oil-based lotion*	
▪ Place 1-2 teaspoons of medication in palm of hand and soften by rubbing briskly between hands.	Softening a topical agent makes it easier to apply to skin.
▪ Once medication is thin and smooth, smear it evenly over skin surface using long even strokes that follow direction of hair growth.	Ensures even distribution of medication. Prevents irritation of hair follicles.
▪ Explain to client that skin may feel greasy after application.	Ointments often contain oils.

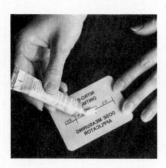

Fig. 72

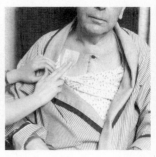

Fig. 73

Steps	Rationale
Antianginal (nitroglycerine) ointment	
▪ Apply desired number of inches of ointment over paper measuring guide. (Fig. 72)	Ensures correct dosage of medication.
▪ (Don disposable glove if desired.) Apply ointment to skin surface by holding edge or back of paper wrapper and placing ointment and wrapper directly on skin. Do not rub or massage ointment into skin. (Fig. 73)	Drug can absorb through your fingertips, causing serious systemic effects. Medication is designed to absorb slowly over several hours and should not be massaged.
▪ Cover ointment and paper with plastic wrap and tape securely (optional).	Prevents soiling of clothing.
Aerosol spray	
▪ Shake container vigorously.	Mixes contents and propellant to ensure distribution of fine even spray.
▪ Read label for distance recommended to hold spray away from area (usually 6-12 inches)	Proper distance ensures that fine spray hits skin surface. Holding container too close results in thin watery distribution.
▪ If neck or upper chest is to be sprayed, ask client to turn face away from spray.	Prevents inhalation of spray.
▪ Spray medication evenly over affected site (in some cases spray is timed for select period of seconds).	Entire affected area of skin should be covered with thin spray.

Steps	Rationale
Suspension-based lotion	
▪ Shake container vigorously.	Mixes powder throughout liquid to form well-mixed suspension.
▪ Apply small amount of lotion to small gauze dressing or pad and apply to skin by stroking evenly in direction of hair growth.	Method leaves protective film of powder on skin after water base of suspension dries. Prevents irritation to hair follicles.
▪ Explain to client that area will feel cool and dry.	Water evaporates to leave thin layer of powder.
Powder	
▪ Be sure that skin surface is thoroughly dry.	Minimizes caking and crusting of powder.
▪ Fully spread apart any skin folds such as between toes or under arms.	Fully exposes skin surface for application.
▪ Dust skin site lightly with dispenser so area is covered with fine thin layer of powder.	Thin layer of powder is more absorbent and reduces friction by increasing area of moisture evaporation (Anders, 1982).
12. Cover skin area with dressing if ordered by physician.	May help prevent agent from being rubbed off skin.
13. Assist client to comfortable position, reapply gown, and cover with bed linen as desired.	Provides for client's sense of well-being.
14. Dispose of soiled supplies in proper receptacle and wash hands.	Keeps client's environment neat and reduces transmission of infection.

Nurse Alert

Assess the client for allergy to topical agents. Avoid patting or rubbing skin when applying creams, ointments, or lotions. This can cause skin irritation. Caution the client against using too much of a medication when performing applications at home. Excess application interferes with drug absorption.

Client Teaching

A client often learns how to apply topical agents at home. Explain the importance of proper hygiene. Caution the client against using too much of a medication since a buildup on the skin interferes with drug absorption. Be sure that the client knows the signs of local reaction to a topical agent.

Pediatric Considerations

When applying topical agents to a young child's skin, it is often necessary to cover the affected area with a dry dressing. Otherwise he may try to rub the medication off.

Geriatric Considerations

The elderly client's skin can be thin and fragile. Apply any topical agent carefully to avoid breaks in the skin. To prevent tape burns, use tape sparingly.

Administering an Eye Medication

The eye is a very sensitive organ. The cornea, or anterior portion of the eyeball, is richly supplied with sensitive pain fibers. The nurse should avoid instilling drops directly onto the corneal surface, so client discomfort will be minimal. It is also important that the nurse use caution in administering eye medications so the applicator does not accidentally touch the eye's surface. Injury can occur easily.

Eye medications are given to dilate the pupil for examination of internal eye structures, to paralyze lens muscles for measurement of lens refraction, to relieve local irritation, to treat eye disorders, and to lubricate the cornea and conjunctiva.

Potential Nursing Diagnoses

Clients who receive eye medications may have one or more of the following nursing diagnoses:

Alteration in sensory perception related to visual disturbance

Potential for injury related to visual alteration

Knowledge deficit regarding drug therapy

Alteration in comfort related to eye infection

Equipment

Prescribed medication with eyedropper or ointment tube
Cotton ball or tissue

Steps	Rationale
1. Review physician's order for name of drug, dose, time of administration, and route.	Ensures safe and accurate administration of drug.
2. Wash your hands.	Reduces transfer of microorganisms.
3. Check client's identification band and ask client's name.	Ensures that right client receives right medication.
4. Explain procedure to client.	Reduces client's anxiety.
5. Ask client to lie supine with neck slightly hyperextended.	Provides easy access to eye for medication instillation. Also minimizes drainage of medication through tear duct.
6. Hold cotton ball or clean tissue in your nondominant hand just below client's lower eyelid. (Fig. 74)	Will absorb any medication that escapes from eye.
7. With tissue resting against client's lower lid margin, gently retract lid downward with your thumb or finger, pressing against bony orbit. *Do not press* directly against eyeball.	Exposes lower conjunctival sac. Retraction against bony orbit prevents pressure and trauma to eyeball.
8. Ask client to look up toward ceiling.	Retracts sensitive cornea up and away from conjunctival sac and reduces stimulation of blink reflex.

Eye Drops

1. Hold eyedropper in your dominant hand approximately 1-2 cm (½-¾ inch) above conjunctival sac. (Fig. 75)	Helps avoid contact of eyedropper with eye structures, thus reducing risk of injury to eye and transfer of infection to dropper.

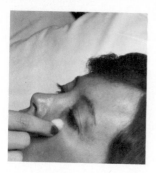

Fig. 74

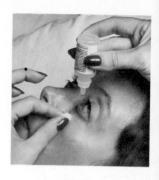

Fig. 75

Steps	Rationale
2. Instill prescribed number of medication drops into conjunctival sac.	Conjunctival sac normally holds 1-2 drops. Applying drops to sac provides for even distribution of medication across eye.
3. If client blinks or closes his eye or if drops land on outer lid margins, repeat procedure.	Therapeutic effect of drug can be obtained only when drops enter conjunctival sac.
4. After instilling drops, ask client to gently close eye.	Helps distribute medication. Squinting or squeezing eyelids forces medication from eyes.
5. When administering drugs that cause systemic effects, protect your finger with clean tissue and apply gentle pressure to client's nasolacrimal duct for 10-15 seconds.	Prevents absorption of medication into systemic circulation.
6. If there is excess medication on eyelids, gently wipe it from inner to outer canthus. If client had an eye patch, apply a clean one.	Promotes client comfort and prevents trauma to eye. Clean patch reduces chances of infection.

Steps	Rationale

Eye Ointment

1. Apply thin stream of ointment evenly along inside edge of lower eyelid, on conjunctiva.

   Serves to distribute medication evenly across eye and lid margin.

2. Have client close his eye and rub lid lightly in circular motion with a cotton ball. NOTE: If client has blepharitis (infection of eyelash follicles), apply ointment to both upper and lower lid margins. Be sure that medication is applied around follicles of both lids.

   Further distributes medication without traumatizing eye.

3. Wash hands and discard supplies.

   Reduces transmission of microorganisms.

4. Record in nurse's notes medication given.

   Timely documentation prevents drug error.

Nurse Alert

To avoid systemic side effects of certain medications, be sure to occlude the nasolacrimal duct (at the inner canthus) after administration.

Client Teaching

It may be necessary to instruct a client who is to receive an eye medication on the technique of self-administration. A client with glaucoma will usually receive medications permanently for control of this disease. Family members should also be taught proper administration techniques, especially after eye surgery when a client's vision is blurred and he has difficulty assembling supplies and handling applicators.

Warn a client against touching eye structures with the applicator. He also should know that preparations are sterile and that they should never be used if prescribed for another family member. It is common for certain medications to cause temporary blurring of vision, and the client should be warned of this.

Pediatric Considerations

A child can easily be frightened when receiving an eye medication. Talk gently with the infant or young child and be sure to restrain his head to prevent movement during instillation. A sudden twist of the head can cause the applicator to accidentally strike the eye. It is also helpful to have the hand that holds the dropper rest on the child's forehead so the hand moves synchronously with the head.

Geriatric Considerations

An elderly client with severe visual alterations will be unable to read labels of prepared medications. Certain clients may learn to recognize containers by their size and shape. However, a family member should be familiar with dose schedules and instillation techniques. A client with motor tremors may not be able to administer drugs safely.

Instilling Ear Drops

Clients receive ear drops to relieve local inflammation and discomfort, soften cerumen, and treat infection. Although ear drops are easy to administer, the nurse should follow three simple safety precautions: instill drops at room temperature to avoid causing vertigo, always use sterile solutions in case the eardrum is ruptured, and avoid instilling ear drops into the ear under pressure.

Potential Nursing Diagnoses

Clients who receive ear drops may have one or more of the following nursing diagnoses:

Sensory alteration related to hearing impairment

Alteration in comfort related to ear inflammation

Knowledge deficit regarding drug therapy and ear disorders

Equipment

Medication dropper
Cotton-tipped applicator
Tissue
Cotton ball (optional)

Steps	Rationale
1. Review physician's order for name of drug, dosage, and route of administration.	Ensures that drug will be safely and accurately administered.
2. Wash hands.	Reduces transfer of microorganisms.

Steps	Rationale
3. Explain procedure to client.	Reduces client anxiety.
4. Check client's identification band and ask client's name.	Ensures right client receives right drug.
5. Have client assume side-lying position with ear to be treated uppermost.	Provides easy access to ear for instillation of medication. Ear canal is in position to retain medication.
6. If cerumen occludes outer portion of ear canal, wipe it out gently with a cotton-tipped applicator. *Do not force wax inward to block or occlude canal.* (Fig. 76)	Cerumen may harbor microorganisms. Its presence blocks distribution of medication into ear canal and can interfere with normal sound conduction.
7. Straighten client's ear canal by pulling pinna down and back (children) or upward and backward (adults). (Fig. 77)	Provides for direct access to deeper external ear structures.
8. Instill prescribed drops, holding dropper 1 cm (½ inch) above ear canal.	Forcing drops into an occluded canal may cause injury to eardrum.

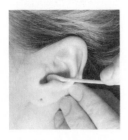

Fig. 76

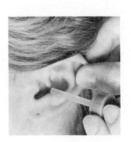

Fig. 77

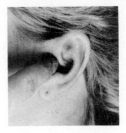

Fig. 78

Steps	Rationale
9. Ask client to remain in side-lying position 2-3 minutes. Apply gentle pressure to tragus of ear with your finger. (Fig. 78)	Allows complete distribution of medication. Pressure on tragus moves medication inward.
10. At times physician will order insertion of portion of a cotton ball into outermost part of ear canal. Do not press cotton into canal. Remove cotton in 15 minutes.	Inserting cotton into outer canal prevents escape of medication when client sits or stands.
11. Wash your hands.	Reduces transfer of microorganisms.
12. Record in medication record drug administered.	Prompt documentation prevents drug errors.

Nurse Alert

If the client has severe pain during instillation of drops, discontinue and report this to the physician.

Client Teaching

During instillation of ear drops the nurse can instruct a client in the proper technique for cleaning the ear canal. Cotton-tipped applicators should not be used because they can compact cerumen. Parents should be warned that young children often place objects in their ears. Thus the parent should know how to inspect the child's ear before instilling drops.

Pediatric Considerations

An infant or young child should be restrained supine with his head turned to the appropriate side. This will prevent him from suddenly moving once the ear dropper is above the ear canal.

Geriatric Considerations

In elderly clients the skin lining the outer ear canal often becomes dry and scaly. This is due to a reduction in sebaceous gland secretion. The drying often results in pruritus.

Instilling Nasal Drops

The most common types of nasal drops are decongestant and antibiotic. The drops can be used to relieve nasal congestion and to treat nasal or sinus irritation. They are easy to administer; however, it is important for the client to be positioned properly so the medication will reach the affected sinus. Potentially serious side effects can occur if nasal drops are used too frequently. The most common side effect is drug rebound; that is, chronic use can irritate the mucosa and cause a worsening of the condition.

Potential Nursing Diagnosis

Clients who receive nasal drops may have one or more of the following nursing diagnoses:

Alteration in comfort related to nasal or sinus irritation
Ineffective breathing pattern related to nasal congestion
Knowledge deficit regarding drug therapy

Equipment

Clean tissue
Prepared medication with dropper
Small pillow (optional)

Steps	Rationale
1. Review physician's order for name of drug, dosage, and route of administration.	Ensures that drug will be administered safely and accurately.
2. Wash hands.	Reduces transmission of microorganisms.

Steps	Rationale
3. Explain procedure to client.	Reduces client anxiety.
4. Check client's identification band and ask client's name.	Ensures that right client receives right medication.
5. Instruct client to blow his nose (unless contraindicated because of risk of increasing intracranial pressure or nose bleeds).	Blowing nose removes mucus and secretions, which block distribution of medication.
6. Ask client to assume a supine position. ▪ To reach posterior pharynx and opening of eustachian tube, tilt client's head backward. ▪ To reach ethmoid or sphenoid sinuses, tilt client's head back over edge of bed or place a small pillow under his shoulder and tilt head back. (Fig. 79, *A*) ▪ To reach frontal and maxillary sinuses, tip client's head back over edge of bed or pillow and turn it toward side to be treated. (Fig. 79, *B*)	Allows medication to drain into affected sinus region. 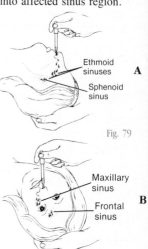 Fig. 79
7. Instruct client to breathe through his mouth.	Reduces chance of aspirating nasal drops into trachea and lungs.
8. Hold dropper 1 cm (½ inch) above naris. Instill the prescribed number of drops toward midline of ethmoid bone.	Dropper becomes contaminated when in contact with mucous membranes. Instilling toward ethmoid bone facilitates distribution of medication over nasal mucosa.

Steps	Rationale
9. Have client remain supine for 5 minutes.	Prevents premature loss of medication through nares.
10. Discard any remaining solution before returning dropper to bottle.	Prevents contamination of remaining medication.
11. Wash your hands.	Reduces transfer of microorganisms.
12. Record in medication record drug administered.	Prompt documentation prevents drug errors.

Client Teaching

Clients should be cautioned about the danger of drug rebound caused by the chronic use of nasal instillations. Encourage clients to follow package directions carefully on any over-the-counter or prescribed nasal preparations.

Pediatric Considerations

Children are positioned the same as adults. However, it may be necessary to gently restrain a child's head. An infant can be held in the nurse's arms with his head extended and stabilized between the nurse's body and elbows.

Geriatric Considerations

An elderly client who experiences nose bleeds should see a physician rather than attempt to treat himself with an over-the-counter preparation. Nose bleeds may merely indicate drying of the mucosa or can be symptomatic of a more serious problem such as hypertension.

Administering
an Inhalant

Drugs given by inhalation are dispersed through an aerosol mist, spray, or fine powder. They are usually designed to produce local effects (for example, dilation of narrowed bronchioles or loosening thick mucus secretions). However, since they are absorbed rapidly through the pulmonary circulation, some drugs have the potential for creating systemic side effects such as cardiac arrhythmias.

Clients with chronic lung disease often depend upon inhalants for control of airway obstruction. Abuse of the medications is a common problem when clients have recurrent symptoms of shortness of breath or dyspnea. Chronic use of over-the-counter inhalants can eventually cause serious side effects.

Potential Nursing Diagnoses

Clients who require use of an inhaled medication may have either or both of the following nursing diagnoses:

Ineffective airway clearance related to tracheobronchial obstruction

Ineffective breathing pattern related to obstruction or inflammation of airways

When the nurse attempts to instruct clients on the use of inhalers, potential diagnoses may include

Knowledge deficit related to drug compliance or inhalant use

Potential noncompliance with drug therapy

Equipment

Metered-dose inhaler with medication canister
Facial tissues (optional)
Wash basin or sink with warm water
Paper towel

Steps	Rationale
1. Allow client an opportunity to manipulate inhaler and canister. Explain and demonstrate how canister fits into inhaler.	Client must be familiar with how to use equipment.
2. Explain what a metered dose is and warn client about overuse of inhaler, including drug side effects.	Client must not arbitrarily decide to administer excessive inhalations due to risk of serious side effects. If drug is given in recommended doses, side effects are uncommon.
3. Explain steps used to administer an inhaled dose of medication (demonstrate steps when possible):	Use of simple step-by-step explanations allows client to ask questions at any point during procedure. You cannot demonstrate actual depression of canister without self-administering a dose.
▪ Remove mouthpiece cover from inhaler.	
▪ With lips open, place inhaler in mouth. Opening should be directed toward back of throat.	
▪ Exhale fully. Then grasp mouthpiece with teeth and lips. (Fig. 80)	Medication should not escape through mouth.
▪ While inhaling slowly and deeply through the mouth, depress medication canister fully.	Medication is distributed to airways during inhalation. Inhalation through mouth draws medication more effectively into airways.

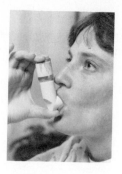

Fig. 80

Steps	Rationale
▪ Hold breath for approximately 10 seconds.	Allows tiny drops of aerosol spray to reach deeper branches of airways.
▪ Then exhale through pursed lips.	Keeps small airways open during exhalation.
4. Instruct client to wait 5-10 minutes between inhalations or as ordered by physician.	Drugs must be inhaled sequentially. First inhalation opens airways and reduces inflammation. Second and third inhalations penetrate deeper airways.
5. Instruct client against repeating inhalations prior to next scheduled dose.	Drugs are prescribed at intervals during day to provide constant bronchodilation and minimize side effects.
6. Explain to client that he may feel sensation in his throat caused by droplets of medication on pharynx or tongue.	Results because inhalant was incorrectly sprayed and inhaled.
7. Instruct client on removing medication canister to clean inhaler. Rinse inhaler in warm water.	Accumulation of spray around mouthpiece can interfere with proper distribution during use.

Steps	Rationale
8. Ask client for any questions.	Provides opportunity to clarify misconceptions or misunderstandings.
9. Have client demonstrate use of inhaler.	Return demonstration provides feedback for measuring client's learning.
10. Record in nurse's notes content or skills taught and client's ability to use inhaler.	Provides continuity to teaching plan so other members of nursing staff will not teach same material.

Nurse Alert

Warn the client that he may gag himself or swallow medication if he fails to inhale while spray is administered.

Client Teaching

Instruct the client on proper use of an inhaler and the common side effects to expect. Explain the common signs and symptoms of xanthine and sympathomimetic drug overuse: tachycardia, palpitations, headache, restlessness, insomnia.

Pediatric Considerations

Children may not be able to learn how to use an inhaler until they reach school age. They also may need to pinch their nose shut during inhalation to gain the drug's effects.

Geriatric Considerations

Elderly clients with hand tremors or weakness in their ability to grasp objects may not be able to use an inhaler.

Instilling a Vaginal Medication

Vaginal medications come in cream and suppository and are used to treat localized infection or inflammation. It is important to avoid embarrassing the client when administering these preparations. Often the client will prefer learning how to self-administer the medication. Because the discharge that is symptomatic of vaginal infections can be foul smelling, it is important to offer good perineal hygiene for the client.

Potential Nursing Diagnoses

Clients who receive vaginal medications may have one or more of the following nursing diagnoses:

Alteration in comfort related to vaginal irritation

Altered self-concept related to vaginal infection

Alteration in health maintenance related to mobility restriction (client unable to self-administer drug)

Knowledge deficit regarding drug therapy

Equipment

Vaginal suppository
Suppository
Clean disposable gloves
Lubricating jelly
Clean tissues
Suppository inserter (optional)
Perineal pad (optional)

Vaginal cream
Cream
Plastic applicator
Clean disposable gloves
Paper towel
Perineal pad (optional)

Steps	Rationale
1. Review physician's order for name of drug, dosage, and route of administration.	Ensures safe and accurate administration of drug.
2. Wash hands.	Reduces risk of transferring microorganisms.
3. Explain procedure to client.	Reduces client anxiety.
4. Check client's identification band and ask client's name.	Ensures that right client receives right medication.
5. Have client lie in dorsal recumbent position.	Provides easy access to and good exposure of vaginal canal. Dependent position of client allows suppository to dissolve in vagina without escaping through orifice.
6. Keep abdomen and lower extremities draped.	Minimizes client embarrassment.
7. Apply disposable gloves.	Prevents transmission of infection between nurse and client.

Suppository

1. Remove suppository from foil wrapper and apply liberal amount of petrolatum jelly to smooth or rounded end. Lubricate gloved index finger of dominant hand.	Reduces friction against mucosal surfaces during insertion.
2. With nondominant gloved hand gently retract labial folds.	Exposes vaginal orifice.
3. Insert rounded end of suppository along posterior wall of vaginal canal length of index finger (7.5 to 10 cm [3 to 4 inches]) (Fig. 81)	Ensures equal distribution of medication along walls of vaginal cavity.

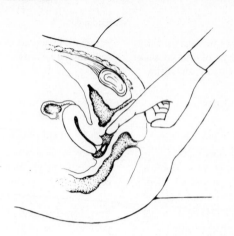

Fig. 81

Steps	Rationale
4. Withdraw finger and wipe away any remaining lubricant from around orifice and labia.	Maintains client comfort.
5. Remove gloves by pulling them inside out and discard them in appropriate receptacle.	Prevents spread of microorganisms.
6. Instruct client to remain on her back for at least 10 minutes.	Allows medication to melt and be absorbed into vaginal mucosa.
7. Offer perineal pad before client resumes ambulation.	Provides for client comfort.
8. Wash hands. NOTE: Follow same procedure when using suppository inserter.	Reduces transfer of microorganisms.
9. Record in medication record drug administered.	Prompt documentation prevents drug errors.

Steps	Rationale
Vaginal Cream	
1. Fill cream applicator, following package directions.	Dosage is prescribed by volume in applicator.
2. With your nondominant gloved hand, gently retract labial folds.	Exposes vaginal orifice.
3. With your dominant gloved hand, insert applicator approximately 7.5 cm (3 inches). Push applicator plunger to deposit medication.	Allows for equal distribution of medication along walls of vaginal cavity.
4. Withdraw plunger and place it on a paper towel. Wipe off any residual cream from labia or vaginal orifice.	Residual cream on applicator may contain microorganisms.
5. Remove gloves and turn them inside out. Dispose of them in appropriate receptacle.	Disposing of gloves in this way reduces transfer of microorganisms.
6. Instruct client to remain flat on her back for at least 10 minutes.	Cream will be distributed and absorbed evenly in vaginal cavity rather than being lost through vaginal orifice.
7. Wash applicator with soap and warm water. Store it for future use.	Vaginal cavity is not sterile. Soap and water will assist in removing bacteria and residual cream.
8. Offer client a perineal pad before she resumes ambulation.	Provides client comfort.
9. Wash your hands.	Reduces transmission of microorganisms.
10. Record in medication record drug administered.	Prompt documentation prevents drug errors.

Client Teaching

Clients often prefer to learn how to self-administer vaginal preparations. Using a step-by-step approach, allow the client to do a demonstration of the technique. It is important that she insert the suppository or cream correctly into the vaginal canal.

Geriatric Considerations

An elderly woman may have difficulty assuming a position that allows for self-administration of vaginal preparations. Arthritic conditions of the hips, knees, or upper extremities can make self-administration painful and difficult.

Inserting a Rectal Suppository

There are various types of drugs available in suppository form that create local as well as systemic effects. Aminophylline suppositories act systemically to dilate the respiratory bronchioles. A Dulcolax suppository acts locally to promote defecation. Suppositories are safe to administer. The nurse should be concerned primarily with placing the suppository correctly against the rectal mucosal wall, past the internal anal sphincter, so the suppository will not be expelled. Clients who have had rectal surgery or who are experiencing rectal bleeding should not be given a suppository.

Potential Nursing Diagnoses

Clients who receive rectal suppositories may have one or more of the following nursing diagnoses:

Alteration in elimination related to constipation and/or fecal impaction

Alteration in health maintenance related to mobility restriction (client unable to self-administer drug)

Knowledge deficit regarding drug therapy

Equipment

Rectal suppository
Lubricating jelly
Clean disposable gloves
Tissue

Steps	Rationale
1. Review physician's order for name of drug, dosage, and route of administration.	Ensures that drug will be administered safely and accurately.
2. Wash hands.	Reduces transfer of microorganisms.
3. Explain procedure to client.	Reduces client anxiety.
4. Check client's identification band and ask client's name.	Ensures that right client receives right medication.
5. Ask client to assume a side-lying (Sims) position with upper leg flexed upward.	Exposes anus and helps client relax external anal sphincter.
6. Keep client draped with only anal area exposed.	Draping client maintains privacy and facilitates relaxation.
7. Remove suppository from its foil wrapper and lubricate rounded end with jelly. Lubricate gloved index finger of your dominant hand.	Lubrication reduces friction as suppository enters rectal canal.
8. Ask client to take slow deep breaths through his mouth and to relax anal sphincter.	Forcing suppository through a constricted sphincter causes pain.
9. Retract client's buttocks with your nondominant hand. With your gloved index finger, insert suppository gently through anus, past internal anal sphincter, and against rectal wall: 10 cm (4 inches) in adults, 5 cm (2 inches) in children and infants. (Fig. 82)	Suppository must be placed against rectal mucosa for eventual absorption and therapeutic action.

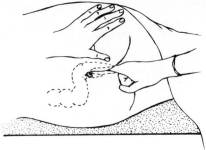

Fig. 82

Steps	Rationale
10. Withdraw your finger and wipe off client's anal area.	Provides client comfort.
11. Discard gloves by turning them inside out and dispose of them in appropriate receptacle.	Disposing of gloves in this way reduces transfer of microorganisms.
12. Instruct client to remain flat or on his side for 5 minutes.	Prevents expulsion of the suppository.
13. If suppository contains a laxative or fecal softener, place call light within client's reach so he can obtain assistance to reach a bedpan or toilet.	Being able to call for assistance provides client with sense of control over elimination.
14. Wash your hands.	Reduces transfer of microorganisms.
15. Record in medication record drug administered.	Prompt documentation prevents drug errors.

Nurse Alert

Although it is unusual, a client may experience a vagal reflex response (slowing of the heart rate) as a result of excessive rectal stimulation.

Client Teaching

Clients may prefer learning how to self-administer rectal suppositories. This can be difficult unless the nurse is clear as to how to insert the suppository past the internal anal sphincter. A client must be familiar with the sensation felt as the sphincter relaxes over the insertion finger.

Pediatric Considerations

The rectal route is chosen only when children are unable to take food or liquid by mouth and when it is unlikely that they have large amounts of stool. The rectum must be empty for effective drug absorption.

Geriatric Considerations

An elderly client may have mobility restrictions that prohibit self-administration of suppositories.

INFECTION
CONTROL

Handwashing

Within a health care environment the risk of infection is ever present. A high population of virulent microorganisms can always be found whenever there have been large numbers of seriously ill clients. Nosocomial infection (resulting from the delivery of health services in a health care facility) is one of the greatest problems in health care today. Hospital-acquired infections resulting from diagnostic or therapeutic procedures often result in extended stays and thus are very costly to clients and health care providers.

Thorough handwashing is the most important and basic technique in preventing and controlling infection. The nurse is constantly handling objects, liquids, or substances contaminated with microorganisms. Unless she washes her hands before and after contact with each client, infection can easily be spread. The Centers for Disease Control (CDC) recommends guidelines for handwashing. Before a nurse begins working with clients a 2-minute handwashing provides good protection. A 30-second hand washing after each routine client contact ensures that the spread of infection will be minimal. Whenever a nurse has handled contaminated equipment or organic material, a 1-minute handwashing is recommended.

Potential Nursing Diagnoses

Nurses perform thorough handwashing before working with all clients. A client at risk of infection due to increased susceptibility from factors such as stress, an open wound, inadequate nutrition, or an altered immune response will require special consideration. He may have any of the following nursing diagnoses:

Potential for injury related to infection

Actual impairment in skin integrity

Alteration in nutrition: less than body requirements

Equipment

Sink with warm running water

Soap or disinfectant in foot-operated dispenser (bar soap may be used)

Paper towels

Orange stick (optional)

Steps	Rationale
1. Push wristwatch and long uniform sleeves up above your wrists. Remove jewelry.	Provides complete access to fingers, hands, and wrists. Jewelry may harbor microorganisms.
2. Keep your fingernails short and filed.	Dirt and secretions that lodge under the fingernails contain microorganisms. Long fingernails can scratch client's skin.
3. Inspect surface of your hands and fingers for any breaks or cuts in skin and cuticles. Report such lesions when caring for highly susceptible clients.	Open cuts or wounds can harbor high concentrations of microorganisms. Such lesions may serve as portals of exit, increasing client's exposure to infection, or as portals of entry, increasing your risk of acquiring an infection.
4. Stand in front of sink, keeping hands and uniform away from sink surface. (If hands touch sink during handwashing, repeat the process.) Use a sink where it is comfortable to reach faucet.	Inside of sink is a contaminated area. Reaching over sink increases risk of touching edge, which is contaminated.

Steps	Rationale
5. Turn on water. Press foot pedals with foot to regulate flow and temperature. Push knee pedals laterally to control flow and temperature. Turn on hand-operated faucets by covering faucet with paper towel.	When hands come in contact with faucet, they are considered contaminated. Organisms spread easily from hands to faucet.
6. Avoid splashing water against your uniform.	Microorganisms travel and grow in moisture.
7. Regulate flow of water so temperature is warm.	Warm water is more comfortable. Hot water opens pores of skin, causing irritation.
8. Wet hands and lower arms thoroughly under running water. Keep hands and forearms lower than elbows during washing. (Fig. 83)	Hands are the most contaminated parts to be washed. Water flows from least to most contaminated area.
9. Apply soap to hands. If bar soap is used, hold it throughout handwashing period. Soap granules, leaflets, and liquid preparations may be used.	Bar soap should be rinsed before return to soap dish. A soap dish that allows water to drain keeps soap firm. Jelly-like soap permits growth of microorganisms.

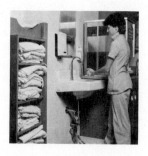

Fig. 83

Steps	Rationale
10. Wash hands using plenty of lather and friction for 15-30 seconds. Interlace fingers and rub palms and back of hands with circular motion. (Fig. 84)	Soap cleanses by emulsifying fat and oil and lowering surface tension. Friction and rubbing mechanically loosen and remove dirt and transient bacteria. Interlacing fingers and thumbs ensures that all surfaces are cleansed.
11. If areas underlying fingernails are soiled, clean them with fingernails of other hand and additional soap or a clean orangewood stick. Do not tear or cut skin under or around nail.	Mechanical removal of dirt and sediment under nails reduces microorganisms on hands.
12. Rinse hands and wrists thoroughly, keeping hands down and elbows up.	Rinsing mechanically washes away dirt and microorganisms.
13. Repeat Steps 9 through 11 but extend actual period of washing for 1-, 2-, and 3-minute handwashings.	Greater the likelihood that hands will be contaminated, greater the need for thorough handwashing.

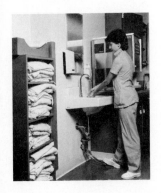

Fig. 84

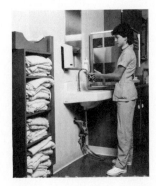

Fig. 85

Steps	Rationale
14. Dry hands thoroughly, wiping from fingers down to wrists and forearms. (Fig. 85)	Dry from cleanest area (fingertips) to least clean (wrists) to avoid contamination. Drying hands prevents chapping and roughened skin.
15. Discard paper towel in proper receptacle.	Proper disposal of contaminated objects prevents transfer of microorganisms.
16. Turn off water with foot and knee pedals. To turn off a hand faucet, use a clean dry paper towel.	Wet towel and wet hands allow transfer of pathogens by capillary action.
17. Keep hands and cuticles well lubricated with hand lotion or moisturizer between washings.	Dry chapped skin cracks easily, creating portal of entry for infection.

Nurse Alert

If the nurse has an open lesion or wound on her hand, some agencies have policies prohibiting her contact with clients.

Care of a Client in Isolation

The nurse must follow special precautions when caring for clients who either have greater susceptibility to infection or are carriers of microorganisms that can be easily transmitted to other persons. Protective isolation or isolation precautions keep the affected client within the confines of his room. The nurse uses protective coverings such as a mask, gown, or gloves depending on how the organism is transmitted and how susceptible the client is to infection. Staying within a confined area and being cared for by nurses covered in protective clothing are factors that can cause a person to feel socially isolated. Whenever the nurse cares for the client in isolation, it is important to maintain therapeutic communication and provide a personalized approach to care.

Potential Nursing Diagnoses

Clients who are placed in protective isolation may have any of the following nursing diagnoses:

Potential for injury related to altered immunity or existing infection

Potential alteration in self-concept related to isolation

Sensory alteration related to isolation status

Equipment

The selection of equipment depends on the type of care to be administered to the client (for example, supplies for administering medications, supplies for hygiene, supplies for bedmaking).

Steps	Rationale
1. Refer to physician's orders for type of isolation in which client is to be placed.	Type of isolation category influences type of protective clothing worn and precautions followed.
2. Refer to policy and procedure manual or infection control policy of institution for precautions to follow.	Each institution may require guidelines that vary from CDC recommendations.
3. Review laboratory test results to determine type of microorganisms for which client is being isolated.	Allows you to know what microorganism is infecting client and medium in which it was identified (e.g., sputum, blood, wound). This information will enable you to be appropriately cautious when handling infected exudate or drainage.
4. Consider types of care measures or procedures to be performed while in client's room.	Helps you anticipate needs for supplies, time your organization while in room, and coordinate your activities.
5. Prepare all necessary equipment and supplies.	Prevents need to leave and reenter room several times, increasing risk of infection.

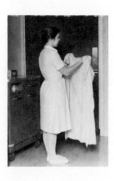

Fig. 86

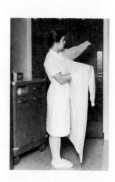

Fig. 87

Steps	Rationale
Donning Protective Clothing	
1. Wash hands.	Reduces transmission of microorganisms.
2. Remove gown from cart. Grasp top of gown at inside with outside facing away from you and allow gown to unfold. (Fig. 86)	Opens gown fully for easier application. Clean gown is not sterile, so you may touch all sides. If gown is reused, outer surface is considered contaminated.
3. Slide your arms forward through sleeves until cuffs cover your wrists. (Fig. 87)	Gown should have long sleeves with tight-fitting cuffs to provide full protection.
4. Pull gown onto and around your shoulders. (Fig. 88)	Gown should completely cover your uniform.
5. Secure ties at neck. (Fig. 89)	Keeps gown in place.
6. Secure ties at your waist.	Prevents gown from falling away from your body, which can cause contamination of your uniform.
7. Put on clean disposable gloves, being sure that edge of glove covers cuff of gown.	Prevents transmission of pathogens by direct and indirect contact.

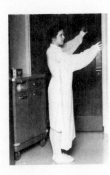

Fig. 88

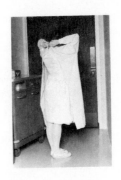

Fig. 89

Steps	Rationale
8. Apply mask securely over your face and mouth (see Skill 5-3).	Protects you from inhaling large-particle aerosols and small-particle droplets. Also protects susceptible clients from organisms that you might spread.

Preparing to Enter Room

1. Leave medication cart or tray outside client's room.	Prevents contamination from repeated transfer in and out of room.
2. Leave brown paper bag and isolation label for specimen collection on isolation cart.	Specimen will eventually be placed in bag, so outer surface of bag remains clean. Thus anyone can transport specimen without fear of contamination.
3. Place stethoscope on inside handle of door or on paper towel away from bedside work area.	Stethoscope should remain free of contamination as you perform care.
4. Avoid taking into room any equipment or supplies that are absolutely essential for use with other clients or by other personnel.	Exposure of equipment to infected material results in contamination. Equipment must be disinfected or sterilized before reuse.

Entering Room

1. Take all necessary equipment and supplies into room. Avoid placing on contaminated surfaces.	Minimizes transmission of microorganisms.
2. Lower glove cuff, remove watch, and place on clean paper towel within easy view.	Wristwatch is used for vital sign measurement and should remain uncontaminated since it is later removed from room.
3. Place specimen containers on clean paper towel in client's bathroom.	Specimen containers will be handled by laboratory personnel. Contamination should be

Steps	Rationale
	kept to minimum. Urine and feces should be transferred in bathroom.

Vital Signs

Steps	Rationale
1. Take stethoscope and place it around neck. During use, be sure that it has minimal contact with contaminated material (e.g., drainage, excretions).	Stethoscope will be reused with other clients and should not contact contaminated material.
2. Measure client's temperature using proper technique (Skills 2-1 to 2-4).	
3. Measure client's blood pressure (Skill 2-7). (Wrap cuff around thin gown sleeve, above antecubital fossa.)	Minimizes contamination of cuff.
4. With watch in view on towel, assess pulse and respirations (Skills 2-5 and 2-6).	If gloved hand touches client or any contaminated object, watch should not be touched.
5. Record results of vital signs on clean paper towel at bedside.	Chart and flow sheets cannot be taken into client's room. You will transcribe results onto form outside room once all care is completed.
6. Place stethoscope on clean surface in room. Wash off diaphragm or bell, if soiled, with alcohol swab.	Stethoscope will be removed from room when nursing care is completed. Alcohol helps disinfect soiled surfaces.

Medications

Steps	Rationale
1. Administer medications using appropriate technique (Skills 4-1 to 4-4, 4-6, and 4-7).	

Steps	Rationale
2. After administering injection, discard contaminated needle and syringe in appropriate containers (e.g., needle cutter) in client's room. Dispose of cups and wrappers in container in room.	Prevents exposure of personnel to contaminated objects by avoiding transport of equipment to medication room.

Specimen Collection

Steps	Rationale
1. Collect necessary specimens using appropriate technique. Transfer specimen to container by minimizing contact of gloved hands with outer surface of container.	Each type of body excretion or exudate must be collected in specific manner to prevent contamination by resident flora. Containers will be handled by laboratory personnel and should remain clean on outside.
2. Be sure that specimen container is sealed tightly.	Prevents spillage and contamination of its outer surface.
3. Label specimen container with client's name.	Properly labeled specimens are essential so correct laboratory results are reported for correct client.
4. Have nurse stand outside client's room holding brown paper bag. Place specimen in bag without contaminating bag's outer surface.	Outer surface of bag is considered clean and can be touched by personnel.
5. Ask second nurse to place isolation label on bag and have specimen transported.	Specimens should be transported to laboratory immediately for proper preparation.

Hygiene (Unit VI)

Steps	Rationale
1. Perform necessary hygiene measures. Avoid allowing gown to become wet.	Moisture on gown provides path for microorganisms to spread to your uniform.

Steps	Rationale
2. Discard soiled linen into special isolation linen bag located in client's room.	Isolation linen bag must be impervious and sturdy to contain contaminated linen.

Bagging Articles

1. If linen bag is filled, be sure that all soiled linen is contained and that top of bag is securely tied. (Fig. 90)	Contaminated linen should be well contained to prevent exposure to health care personnel.
2. Have second nurse stand outside client's room and hold clean linen bag. (Fig. 91)	Double bagging prevents exposure of personnel to contaminated outer surface of soiled linen bag.
3. Nurse outside room holds clean bag by folding its top edges back to form a cuff over her hands.	Cuff protects you from contacting soiled linen bag.
4. As opening of bag separates, place your hand inside clean bag and pull opening out fully.	Inside of bag is considered contaminated. Outer bag should be opened so contaminated bag can be easily dropped in.

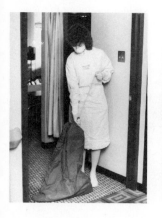

Fig. 90

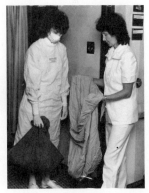

Fig. 91

Steps	Rationale
5. Drop contaminated linen bag into clean receiving bag without touching receiving bag's sides. (Fig. 92)	Contaminated bag is contained and can now be transported outside client's room.
6. Have second nurse discard linen into appropriate hamper.	Institutional policy may vary as to where to dispose of isolation linen.
7. Take any contaminated reusable objects (e.g., suction bottles or instruments) and carefully place in paper or plastic bag held by second nurse outside room.	CDC recommends single bag as adequate to discard items if bag impervious and sturdy and article can be placed inside it without contaminating outer surface. Otherwise, follow double-bag procedure.
8. Second nurse seals bag with tape or according to agency policy.	Contains contaminated item safely.

Preparing To Leave Room

1. Be sure that client's needs have been attended to.	Attempt to minimize number of visits into isolation room, particularly when strict precautions are being followed. You may not return to room for some time.

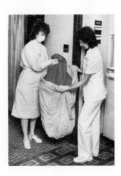

Fig. 92

Steps	Rationale
2. Remove gloves by grasping cuff of one glove and pulling it off, turning glove inside out. With your ungloved hand, tuck finger inside cuff of remaining glove and pull off, turning inside out. Dispose of it in proper receptacle.	Gloves are removed first since they are most likely to be contaminated and should not be used to touch hair around mask.
3. Untie or pull off mask from around your ears and dispose of it in receptacle.	Masks are disposable.
4. Untie gown from around your neck and waist. Keeping your hand inside one cuff, pull opposite sleeve down from arm. Do same for other arm.	Keeping hands inside gown minimizes contact with microorganisms.
5. Pull gown off by turning it inside out. Fold so contaminated sides face one another. Discard in proper receptacle.	Gown is turned inside out so hands and clothing do not come in contact with contaminated outer surface.
6. Wash your hands thoroughly.	Mechanically removes any transient microorganisms contacted.
7. Pick up wristwatch and stethoscope, taking care not to touch a contaminated surface. Note vital sign recordings made in room.	Clean hands may touch watch and stethoscope.
8. Leave room, closing door securely.	Room should remain closed, especially when airborne infection is being isolated.
9. Record in nurse's notes vital signs and other procedures according to guidelines for each skill.	Documents care provided.

Nurse Alert

Be sure that you are familiar with the specific guidelines for each isolation category. It is important to know what type of infection the client has and in what manner the infective organisms are transmitted.

Client Teaching

Explain the purpose for and importance of isolation techniques. Clients must understand that the precautions used are for everyone's safety. If the client understands isolation practices, he can help enforce procedures when visitors enter the room.

Pediatric Considerations

Preschoolers may view isolation as a form of punishment. Older children should be given a thorough explanation of procedures to minimize fears and fantasies. Show children the different forms of protective clothing. Young children can play "dress up" with masks and gloves. If possible, allow children to see your face before applying a mask.

Geriatric Considerations

Elderly clients may be more at risk than younger clients of sensory deprivation due to normal processes. They will consistently need meaningful sensory stimuli while in isolation. Some simple actions to take might include turning on the lights when entering the room, raising the head of the bed and repositioning the client, opening window shades or curtains, and sitting down to have a relaxed discussion.

Donning a Surgical Mask

A mask may be worn for several reasons: as a precaution to reduce air-droplet transmission of microorganisms while caring for a client in isolation, when assisting with a sterile procedure, or when preparing sterile supplies for a sterile field. The nurse should apply the mask snugly around face and nose; otherwise it is ineffective in controlling air-droplet nuclei. A mask is always applied before the nurse performs a surgical handwash. When a mask becomes moist, it should be changed. Moisture promotes the spread of microorganisms.

Potential Nursing Diagnoses

The nurse will apply a mask when caring for clients with a variety of nursing diagnoses. However, clients with the following diagnosis require special precautions:

Potential for injury related to infection

Equipment

Clean disposable mask

Steps	Rationale

Application of Mask

1. Find top edge of mask (usually has a thin metal strip along edge).

   Pliable metal fits snugly against bridge of nose.

2. Hold mask by top two strings or loops. Tie two top ties at the top of the back of your head, with ties *above* your ears (alternative: slip loops over each ear). (Fig. 93)

   Position of ties at top of head provides tight fit. Ties over ears may cause irritation.

3. Tie two lower ties snugly around your neck, with mask well under chin. (Fig. 94)

   Prevents escape of microorganisms through sides of mask as you talk or breathe.

4. Gently pinch upper metal band around the bridge of your nose.

   Prevents microorganisms from escaping around nose.

Removal of Mask

1. If you have gloves on, remove them and wash your hands.

   Prevents contamination of hair, neck, and face from contact with soiled gloves.

2. Untie both ties and fold mask in half with inner surfaces together.

   Avoids contact with contaminated inner surface.

3. Dispose of mask in receptacle.

   Reduces spread of infection.

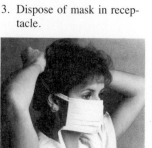

Fig. 93

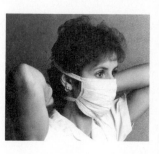

Fig. 94

Nurse Alert

In the operating room, apply a second mask over the first once the first mask becomes moist. Removal of a mask in the surgical area causes immediate contamination of surrounding objects.

Client Teaching

When caring for a client in isolation, explain the purpose of a mask. The mask may add to a client's feeling of becoming depersonalized.

Pediatric Considerations

If a child is awake in the operating room, allow him to see your face, if possible, before applying the mask.

Surgical Handwashing

Nurses who work in sterile areas such as the operating room or labor and delivery rooms must practice surgical handwashing. The technique requires greater effort than routine handwashing. During a surgical scrub the nurse washes a wider area, from fingertips to elbows. Usually the duration of a scrub lasts 5 to 10 minutes to ensure that all skin surfaces are thoroughly cleaned. For maximal cleansing and removal of bacteria the nurse removes all jewelry from her fingers and arms and keeps her fingernails short, clean, and free of polish.

Potential Nursing Diagnoses

This procedure, designed to minimize the presence of microorganisms on the nurse's hands, may be done by anyone caring for clients who have the following nursing diagnosis:

Potential for injury related to infection

Equipment

Deep sink with foot pedals or knee controls.
Antiseptic detergent in a foot-controlled dispenser
Hand brushes
Orange stick or disposable nail file

Steps	Rationale
1. Check hands and fingers for cuts or abrasions	Areas of inflammation or breaks in skin can harbor microorganisms.

Steps	Rationale
2. Remove all jewelry.	Harbors microorganisms.
3. Apply a face mask, making certain to cover your nose and mouth snugly.	Prevents escape of microorganisms into air, which can contaminate hands.
4. Adjust water flow to lukewarm temperature.	Hot water removes protective oils from the skin and increases skin's sensitivity to soap.
5. Wet your hands and forearms liberally, keeping hands above level of elbows during entire procedure. NOTE: Your scrub dress or uniform must be kept dry.	Water runs by gravity from fingertips to elbows. Hands become cleanest part of upper extremity. Keeping hands elevated allows water to flow from least to most contaminated area.
6. Dispense a liberal amount of soap (2-5 ml) into hands and lather hands and arms to 5 cm (2 inches) above elbows.	Washing wide area reduces risk of contaminating overlying gown that you will apply.
7. Clean nails with orange stick or file under running water. (Fig. 95)	Removes dirt and organic material that harbor large numbers of microorganisms.

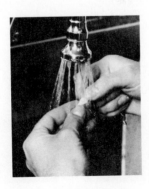

Fig. 95

Steps	Rationale
8. Rinse hands and arms thoroughly, keeping your hands above level of elbows.	Removes transient bacteria from fingers, hands, and forearms.
9. Lather your hands and arms and scrub each hand with brush for 45 seconds. Using same brush, scrub each arm to 5 cm (2 inches) above elbow. Divide arm into thirds: scrub each lower forearm 15 seconds, each upper forearm 15 seconds, and 5 cm above each elbow 15 seconds. (Fig. 96)	Scrubbing loosens resident bacteria that adhere to skin's surface.
10. Discard brush and rinse your hands and arms thoroughly.	After touching skin, brush is considered contaminated. Rinsing removes resident bacteria.
11. Using second brush, scrub each hand for 30 seconds. Use same brush to scrub each arm up to elbow. Divide arm in half: scrub each lower forearm 15 seconds and each upper forearm 15 seconds.	Second scrubbing ensures thorough cleaning of hands and forearms. Number of resident microorganisms remaining on skin will be minimal.

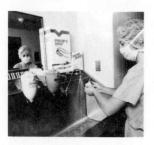

Fig. 96

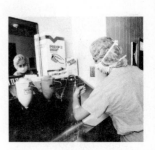

Fig. 97

Steps	Rationale
12. Discard brush and rinse your hands and arms thoroughly. Turn off water with foot pedal. (Fig. 97)	Prevents contamination of hands.
13. Use sterile towel to dry one hand thoroughly, moving from fingers to elbow. Dry in a rotating motion. NOTE: If you wish to apply sterile gloves for use in a regular clinical area you need not use brushes or dry your hands with sterile towels. Thorough lathering and friction performed twice according to procedure will ensure clean hands. In this situation you may use clean paper towels for drying.	Dry from cleanest to least clean area. Drying prevents chapping and facilitates donning of gloves.
14. Repeat drying method for other hand, using different area of towel or a new sterile towel.	Prevents contamination of hand.
15. Keep hands higher than elbows and away from your body.	Prevents accidental contamination.
16. Proceed into operating room or labor and delivery area, keeping hands from contacting any object.	If your hands touch any object, scrub must be repeated.

Nurse Alert

Throughout the procedure and afterwards the nurse must not allow an unsterile object to touch her hands or lower arms.

Donning a Sterile Gown

The nurse must wear a sterile gown in the operating room and delivery room so sterile objects can be comfortably handled with less risk of contamination. Nurses assisting physicians with invasive procedures in a treatment room may also wear sterile gowns. A gown is applied after surgical handwashing and after the nurse has donned a mask and surgical cap. She either picks up the gown from a sterile field or has a gowned assistant hand her one.

The entire surface of the gown is not considered sterile. Only the area from the anterior waist to, but not including, the collar and anterior surface of the sleeves is sterile.

Potential Nursing Diagnoses

This procedure may be performed by nurses caring for clients with a variety of nursing diagnoses.

Equipment

Disposable mask
Disposable cap
Sterile gown (prepared for donning by circulating nurse)

Steps	Rationale
1. Don mask and cap. Carry out surgical handscrubbing for at least 5 minutes.	Scrubbing eliminates microorganisms from surface of hands. Mask and cap reduce chances of transmitting organisms to gown by direct contact and airborne transmission.
2. Pick up gown, grasping inside surface at collar. (Fig. 98)	Hands are not completely sterile. Inside surface of gown will contact skin surface and is thus considered contaminated.
3. Stand away from sterile pack and table. Hold gown at arm's length away from your body and allow gown to unfold by itself. Be careful not to allow gown to touch floor.	Contact of outer surface of gown with a dirty or clean surface would result in gown contamination. Shaking of gown can cause air currents that increase risk of contamination.
4. Hold gown by inside, open shoulder seams, and insert each hand through armholes. (Fig. 99)	Inside surface of gown is considered contaminated.

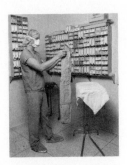

Fig. 98

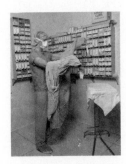

Fig. 99

Steps	Rationale
5. Keeping your upper arms in front of you at shoulder height, extend hands toward gown cuff. (Do not push hands through cuffs if using closed glove method.)	Extension of arms straight ahead keeps sterile outer surface of gown in view and reduces risk of touching floor or a portion of your body.
6. Have circulating nurse assist by reaching inside gown and pulling inner shoulder and side seams onto your shoulders.	Working from behind scrub nurse prevents contamination by circulating nurse. Gown should fit comfortably.
7. Have circulating nurse tie or snap gown at neckline and waist. Only ties or snaps should be touched. (Fig. 100)	Provides secure fit without contamination.
8. If gown is a wraparound style, enclose waist tie or snap in front with a sterile towel. (Keep your hands inside sleeves while grasping towel.) Hand sterile towel to circulating nurse.	Towel provides a surface that circulating nurse can grasp without contaminating gown.

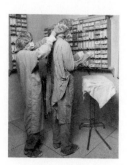

Fig. 100

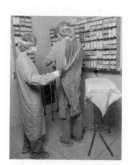

Fig. 101

Steps	Rationale
9. Circulating nurse grasps edge of towel without touching tie while you pivot in opposite direction from her. (Fig. 101)	Wraparound gown achieves better coverage of your body and reduces risk of contamination.
10. Take tie from towel wrapper, keeping your hands inside sleeves, and tie gown in front. Make certain that gown is completely closed.	Gown must be securely tied while worn in operating room.

Nurse Alert

If the gown comes in contact with any unsterile object, including the nurse's hands, it is considered to be contaminated.

Open Gloving

The nurse applies sterile gloves by the open method when preparing to work with certain types of sterile equipment and when performing sterile procedures such as dressing changes or catheter insertion. The gloves provide a barrier between the nurse's hands and the objects she contacts. She is able to freely touch objects in a sterile field without concern of contamination. When wearing sterile gloves, she should always remain conscious of which objects are sterile and which are not. A glove becomes contaminated whenever it contacts a nonsterile object.

Potential Nursing Diagnoses

The nurse will use sterile gloves while caring for clients who have any of a number of nursing diagnoses. However, the following requires special precautions:

Potential for injury related to infection

Equipment

Package of sterile gloves of proper size

Steps	Rationale
1. Wash hands thoroughly.	Reduces numbers of microorganisms residing on surfaces of hands.
2. Remove outer package wrapper by carefully peeling apart sides.	Prevents inner glove package from accidentally opening and touching contaminated objects.

Steps	Rationale
3. Grasp inner package and lay it on a clean flat surface just above waist level. Open package, keeping gloves on wrapper's inside surface.	Sterile object held below your waist is considered contaminated. Inner surface of glove package is considered sterile.
4. If gloves are not prepowdered, take packet of powder and apply lightly to hands over a sink or wastebasket.	Powder allows gloves to slip on easily. (Some physicians do not use powder for fear of promoting growth of microorganisms).
5. Identify right and left glove. Each glove has a cuff approximately 5 cm (2 inches) wide. Glove your dominant hand first.	Proper identification of gloves prevents contamination by improper fit. Gloving of dominant hand first improves your dexterity with procedure.
6. With thumb and first two fingers of your nondominant hand, grasp edge of cuff of glove for dominant hand. Touch only the glove's inside surface. (Fig. 102)	Inner edge of cuff will lie against your skin and thus is not considered sterile. NOTE: Left hand dominant in photo.
7. Carefully pull glove over your dominant hand, leaving a cuff and being sure that cuff does not roll up your wrist. Be	If glove's outer surface touches your hand or wrist, it is contaminated.

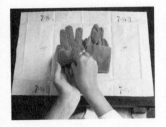

Fig. 102

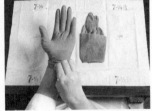

Fig. 103

Steps	Rationale
sure also that thumb and fingers are in proper spaces. (Fig. 103)	
8. With your gloved dominant hand, slip your fingers underneath second glove's cuff. (Fig. 104)	Cuff protects your gloved fingers. Sterile touching sterile prevents glove contamination.
9. Carefully pull second glove over your nondominant hand. Do not allow fingers and thumb of gloved dominant hand to touch any part of your exposed nondominant hand. Keep thumb of dominant hand abducted back. (Fig. 105)	Contact of gloved hand with exposed hand results in contamination.

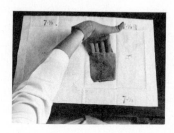

Fig. 104

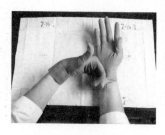

Fig. 105

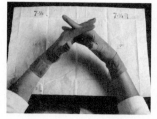

Fig. 106

Steps	Rationale
10. Once second glove is on, interlock your hands. Cuffs usually fall down after application. Be sure to touch only sterile sides. (Fig. 106)	Ensures smooth fit over fingers.

Nurse Alert

If the outer (clean) surface of a glove touches a nonsterile object, such as a portion of your arm or the table surface, remove and repeat gloving.

Client Teaching

Explain to the client why gloves are used during a procedure. At times the client may perceive the use of gloves as the nurse's reluctance to touch him.

Closed Gloving

The technique of closed gloving is used primarily by nurses who work in sterile treatment areas such as the operating room or labor and delivery rooms. Closed gloving differs from open gloving in that the nurse's hands are kept covered by a sterile gown cuff throughout the procedure. Placement of each glove over a gown cuff provides added protection against contamination.

Potential Nursing Diagnoses

When working with clients in a sterile area, the nurse is always at risk of infection since the clients usually are undergoing invasive procedures. A nursing diagnosis might include the following:

Potential for injury related to infection

Equipment

Package of sterile gloves of correct size

Steps	Rationale
1. Don a sterile gown (according to Skill 5-5) after thorough handwashing.	Closed gloving is performed only after a sterile gown has been put on.
2. Have circulating nurse open glove package.	You can then easily pick up and apply gloves. Remember, you will be wearing sterile gown and cannot prepare gloves without contaminating gown.

Steps	Rationale
3. Keep your scrubbed hands within sleeve of surgical gown at point of cuff seams.	Prevents your bare hands from contacting sterile exterior of gown.
4. Grasp inside of cuff sleeve covering your nondominant hand. With same hand, pick up glove for your dominant hand. Place glove palm side down on palm of covered dominant hand. Have glove fingers pointing toward elbow of dominant arm. (Fig. 107)	Gown protects your fingers. Sterile touching sterile is sterile. Positioning of glove will allow you to slip it over gown cuff.
5. Fingers of your covered dominant hand pinch underside of glove's cuff. With your covered nondominant hand, grasp topside of glove's cuff for dominant hand. Pull glove over gown cuff and fingers of dominant hand simultaneously. (Fig. 108)	Since your fingers do not exit through gown's cuff, gown and glove contamination is prevented.
6. Carefully push your fingers into glove and be sure glove's cuff covers gown's cuff.	Ensures proper fit. Glove fits over gown cuff to provide extra protection against contamination.

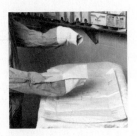

Fig. 107

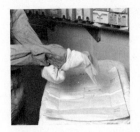

Fig. 108

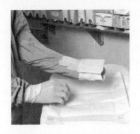

Fig. 109

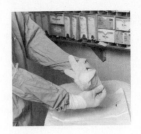

Fig. 110

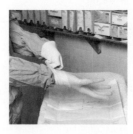

Fig. 111

Steps	Rationale
7. With your gloved dominant hand, place opposite glove palm side down over palm of your covered nondominant hand, glove fingers toward elbow. (Fig. 109)	Sterile touching sterile is sterile.
8. Repeat Steps 5 and 6 for nondominant hand. (Figs. 110, 111)	
9. Interlock gloved hands.	Ensures smooth fit over fingers.

Nurse Alert

If the glove contacts any nonsterile object, it is considered contaminated and the procedure must be repeated.

Giving a Bed Bath

There are several types of baths, classified by the level of assistance that the client requires. A nurse administers a bed bath to clients who are physically dependent for at least a portion of their care. Clients should be encouraged to do as much as possible for themselves during the bath. While providing a bed bath, the nurse has an excellent opportunity to actively interact with the client and conduct physical assessment.

A bed bath stimulates circulation to the skin, promotes cleanliness and control of body odors, provides exercise through joint range of motion, and induces relaxation and comfort.

Potential Nursing Diagnoses

Clients in need of a bed bath may have one or more of the following nursing diagnoses:

Self-care deficit: bathing
Potential alteration in skin integrity
Actual alteration in skin integrity
Reduced activity tolerance
Impaired physical mobility

Equipment

Two bath towels, one for face and one for body
Two washcloths
Washbasin with water temperature adjusted for client's comfort (43° to 46° C, 110° to 115° F)
Soap and soap dish
Bath blanket to cover client during bath

Clean gown or pair of pajamas
Additional bed linens if required
Hygienic aids: powder, deodorant, skin lotion, antiperspirant
Bedpan or urinal
Linen hamper or laundry bag

Steps	Rationale
1. Review client's chart for orders or specific precautions concerning movement and positioning.	Ensures safety of both you and client as well as promotes use of good body mechanics for your protection during procedure.
2. Explain bathing procedure, assess client's physical ability to assist with bath, and determine client's preferences for hygiene practices.	Provides for client's cooperation and participation. Involvement of client in planning bath promotes client independence and results in a plan consistent with his hygiene habits.
3. Assemble equipment and arrange it for convenience on bedside and overbed stand. Remove all unnecessary equipment such as call light or water pitcher.	Planning and assembling equipment permit smooth flow of procedure. This contributes to efficiency and enhances client comfort.
4. Adjust room temperature and ventilation. Make sure all doors and windows are closed to prevent drafts.	Warm room prevents rapid loss of body heat during bathing.
5. Provide privacy by drawing curtain or closing door.	Ensuring client's mental comfort is as important as ensuring his physical comfort.
6. Offer bedpan or urinal.	Client will feel more comfortable after voiding, and interruption of bath may be avoided.
7. Wash your hands.	Reduces transmission of microorganisms.

Steps	Rationale
8. Lower side rail and assist client to a comfortable position, maintaining body alignment.	Client comfort is maintained throughout procedure.
9. Bring client toward side closest to you. Place bed in high position.	When you do not have to reach across bed, strain on your back muscles is minimized.
10. Loosen top covers at foot of bed. Fold and remove top sheet from underneath. If possible, have client hold bath blanket while you withdraw top sheet. If client is unable to hold blanket, hold bath blanket with one hand while removing top sheet with other.	Removal of top linens prevents their becoming soiled or moist during bath. Blanket provides warmth and privacy.
11. If top sheet is to be reused, fold it for replacement. If not, dispose of it in laundry bag, taking care not to allow linen to come in contact with your uniform.	Proper disposal prevents transmission of microorganisms.
12. Remove client's gown or pajamas. If an extremity is injured, begin removal from *uninjured* side. If client has an intravenous tube, remove gown from arm *without* IV first, then lower IV container and slide gown over IV tubing and over IV container. Rehang IV container and check flow rate. (Figs. 112, 113, 114, 115)	Removal of gown allows full exposure of body parts during bathing. Undressing unaffected side first allows easier manipulation of gown over body part with reduced range of motion.

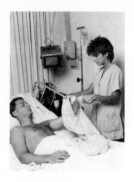

Fig. 112

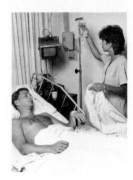

Fig. 113

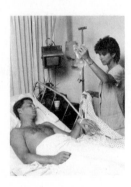

Fig. 114

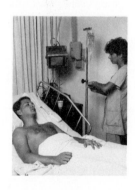

Fig. 115

Steps	Rationale
13. Pull side rails up. Fill washbasin two thirds full with water between 43° and 46°C warm (110° and 115° F). Keep water and room temperatures at comfortable level.	Side rails maintain client's safety as you leave bedside. Warm water promotes comfort and prevents unnecessary chilling.
14. If allowed, remove pillow and raise head of bed 30 degrees. Place a bath towel under client's head. (Some clients, e.g., those	Pillow removal makes it easier to wash client's ears and neck. Placement of a bath towel under head prevents bed linen from becoming wet.

Steps	Rationale
with breathing difficulties, require a pillow or head of bed elevated at all times.)	
15. Make a mitt with washcloth. (Fig. 116)	Mitt retains water and heat better than a loosely held washcloth, keeps cold edges from rubbing against client, and prevents splashing.
16. Place a face towel over client's chest.	Prevents soiling of bath blanket.
17. Wash client's eyes without soap, using a different section of mitt for each eye. Move mitt from inner toward outer canthus. Do not apply direct pressure to eyes. Encrustations on eyelids may re-	Soap irritates eyes. Use of separate sections of mitt prevents spread of microorganisms. Bathing from inner to outer canthus prevents secretions from entering nasolacrimal ducts. Pressure over eyes can cause internal injury.

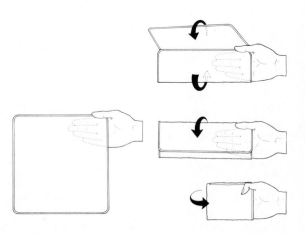

Fig. 116

Steps	Rationale
quire soaking before removal. Dry eyes thoroughly.	
18. Ask client if he prefers soap used on his face. Wash, rinse, and dry his forehead, cheeks, nose, neck, and ears. (Men may wish to shave either at this point or after the bath.)	Soap tends to dry on face more quickly since face is exposed to air more than other parts of body.
19. Expose arm farther from you and place bath towel lengthwise under it.	By bathing farther side first, you avoid having to reach over a clean area. Towel protects bed from becoming wet.
20. Bathe arm with soap and water using long firm strokes from distal to proximal areas. Raise and support arm above the head (if possible) while washing axilla thoroughly.	Soap lowers surface tension and facilitates removal of debris and bacteria when friction is applied during washing. Long firm strokes stimulate circulation. Movement of arm above head exposes axilla for thorough cleaning and facilitates normal range of motion.
21. Rinse and dry arm and underarm well. If client uses deodorant or talcum powder, apply it.	Moisture can cause skin maceration (excessive softening).
22. Fold towel in half and place basin on it so client's hand can be immersed in water.	
23. Allow client's hand to soak for a few minutes before washing it and fingernails in basin. Clean and trim nails if necessary. Remove basin and dry hand well.	Soaking hands softens cuticles and loosens debris beneath nails; it helps client feel his hands are really clean. Drying hands well removes moisture from between fingers.

Steps	Rationale
Repeat Steps 20 to 23 for opposite arm.	
24. Cover client's chest with bath towel and fold bath blanket down to client's umbilicus.	Prevents unnecessary exposure of body parts.
25. With one hand, lift edge of towel away from client's chest. With mitted hand, bathe his chest using long firm strokes. Take special care to wash skinfolds under female client's breasts. It may be necessary to lift each breast while doing this. Keep client's chest covered between wash and rinse periods.	Towel maintains warmth and privacy. Firm strokes stimulate circulation and help prevent chilling. Secretions and dirt collect in skinfolds.
26. Place bath towel lengthwise over abdomen. Fold blanket down to pubic region.	Prevents unnecessary exposure of body parts.
27. With one hand lift bath towel. With mitted hand bathe client's abdomen, giving special attention to umbilicus and abdominal folds. Stroke from side to side. Keep abdomen covered between washing and rinsing. Dry well.	Moisture and sediment that collect in skinfolds predispose client to skin maceration and irritation.
28. Expose far leg by folding bath blanket over toward client's midline. Drape perineum.	Prevents unnecessary exposure.
29. Bend client's leg at knee by positioning your arm under leg. While grasping client's heel, elevate his leg from mattress slightly	Towel protects bed linen from wetness. Support of joint and extremity during lifting prevents strain on musculoskeletal structures.

Steps	Rationale
and slide bath towel lengthwise under it.	
30. Place basin on a towel on bed and secure its position near foot to be washed.	
31. With one hand supporting leg, raise leg and slide basin under lifted foot. Make sure that foot is firmly placed on bottom of basin. Let foot soak while you wash leg.	Position foot to avoid pressure from edge of basin on calf. Soaking softens calluses and rough skin.
32. Use long, smooth, firm strokes, washing from ankle to knee and from knee to thigh. Dry well.	Promotes venous return.
33. Clean foot, making sure to bathe between toes. Clean and clip nails as needed. Dry well. If skin is dry, apply lotion.	Secretions and moisture may be present in skinfolds between toes. Lotion helps to retain moisture and soften skin.

Repeat Steps 28 to 33 for the other foot.

Steps	Rationale
34. Cover client with bath blanket and change bath water. Remember to raise side rails for client safety.	Drop in water temperature during bath can cause chilling. Clean water reduces microorganisms transmission.
35. Help client to a prone or side-lying position. Place a towel lengthwise along his side.	Provides access to back and buttocks.
36. Cover client by sliding bath blanket down from shoulder to thighs and tuck securely under thighs.	Maintains warmth and prevents unnecessary exposure.
37. Wash, rinse, and dry back from neck to but-	Skinfolds near buttocks and anus may contain fecal secre-

Steps	Rationale

tocks using long firm strokes. Pay special attention to folds of buttocks and anus. / tions that harbor microorganisms.

38. Change water and washcloth. / Prevents transfer of microorganisms from anal area to genitalia.

39. Assist client to a supine or side-lying position. Cover chest and upper extremities with a towel and lower extremities with bath blanket. Expose only genitalia. (If client can assist, covering entire body with bath blanket is preferable.) Wash, rinse, and dry perineum (see Skills 6-4 and 6-5), giving special attention to skinfolds. (Allow client to bathe himself if able.) / Maintains client's privacy.

40. Apply body lotion or oil to moisturize skin, if desired. / Prevents dry chapped skin.

41. Assist client in dressing as needed.

42. Comb client's hair; women may want to apply makeup.

43. Make client's bed (see Skill 6-15).

44. Clean and replace bathing equipment. Replace call light and personal possessions. Leave room as comfortable as possible. / A clean environment promotes client comfort. Keeping call light and articles of care within reach promotes client safety.

45. Wash your hands. / Reduces microorganism transmission.

Steps	Rationale
46. Report and record on client's chart any significant findings or abnormal data such as reddened skin areas or joint or muscle pain on movement. Record level of assistance required by client.	Timely documentation maintains accuracy of client's record.

Nurse Alert

Monitor the client's level of fatigue. It may become necessary to discontinue the bath and resume it at a later time.

Client Teaching

Bathing is an excellent time to explain the advantages of good hygiene. During the bath the nurse may observe skin lesions that will require special instructions or care.

Pediatric Considerations

An infant may be given a sponge bath or be bathed in a washbasin. Care is taken to keep the infant covered as much as possible during the procedure to prevent temperature loss. A bath can be a pleasant time for the infant or child because of meaningful tactile stimulation.

Geriatric Considerations

An elderly client's skin will normally be drier and less elastic than that of a younger client. A daily bath is therefore not necessary. It may also be unnecessary to use soap on the older client's skin. Liberal amounts of body lotion will achieve needed lubrication. Give the client time to change positions slowly.

Assisting a Client with a Tub Bath or Shower

For clients who are relatively independent and mobile a tub bath or shower provides a more thorough means of cleaning the skin. A tub bath enables the client to immerse himself in water and thus more easily clean less accessible body parts. A shower is ideal for the client who is active but who cannot immerse the entire body (such as a person with a lower leg cast or dressing).

The most important concern of the nurse is to ensure the client's safety. A wet tub or shower is quite slippery. The nurse must take precautions to prevent falls.

Potential Nursing Diagnoses

Clients who take a tub bath or shower may have one or more of the following nursing diagnoses in relation to hygienic needs:

Potential alteration in skin integrity
Actual alteration in skin integrity
Potential for injury related to risk of falling

Equipment

Two bath towels
Two washcloths
Soap
Hygienic aids: powder, deodorant, skin lotion
Clean gown or pair of pajamas
Slippers and robe

Steps	Rationale
1. Schedule use of bathtub or shower if client does not have private bathroom.	Prevents unnecessary waiting that can fatigue client.
2. Check tub or shower to determine if it needs cleaning. Use cleaning techniques according to agency policy. Place rubber mat on bottom of tub or shower. Place a disposable bath mat or towel on floor in front of tub or shower.	Cleaning prevents transmission of infection. Mats prevent slipping and falling.
3. Collect necessary equipment and place it within easy reach of tub or shower.	Placing items close at hand prevents possible falls when client reaches for equipment.
4. Assist client to bathroom if necessary. Have client wear a robe and slippers en route to bathroom.	Assistance prevents accidental falls. Robe and slippers prevent chilling.
5. Demonstrate to client how to use call signal for assistance.	Bathrooms are equipped with signaling devices in case client feels faint or weak and needs immediate assistance.
6. Place an "occupied" sign on bathroom door.	Maintains client's privacy.
7. Fill bathtub halfway with warm water (41° C, 105.8° F). Ask client to test water. Adjust temperature if too warm. Explain which faucet controls hot water. If client is taking shower, turn shower on and adjust water temperature before client enters shower stall.	Adjusting temperature prevents accidental burns.

Steps	Rationale
8. Instruct client to use safety bars when getting in and out of tub or shower.	Prevents slipping or falls.
9. Instruct client not to remain in tub longer than 20 minutes. Check on client every 5 minutes.	Prolonged exposure to warm water may cause vasodilation and pooling of blood, leading to light-headedness or dizziness.
10. Return to bathroom when client signals and knock before entering.	
11. For client who is unsteady, drain tub of water before client attempts to get out.	Prevents accidental falls.
12. Assist client out of tub as necessary and help with drying.	Moisture may cause maceration of skin and promote spread of infection.
13. Assist client as needed in donning clean gown or pajamas, slippers, and robe.	Maintains warmth to prevent chilling.
14. Assist client to his room and help him assume comfortable position in bed or chair.	Maintains relaxation gained from bathing.
15. Clean tub or shower according to agency policy. Remove soiled linen and place it in dirty linen bag. Discard any disposable equipment in proper receptacle. Place an ''unoccupied'' sign on bathroom door. Return supplies to storage area.	Prevents transmission of microorganisms through soiled linen and moisture.
16. Wash your hands.	Reduces transmission of microorganisms.

Steps	Rationale
17. Record and report client's response to bath or shower and condition of client's skin.	Timely recording provides accurate documentation.

Nurse Alert

Observe the client closely for signs of a drop in blood pressure (dizziness, etc.) due to vasodilation. This is common in clients who have been on bedrest and are taking a bath or shower for the first time.

Client Teaching

The nurse may use this opportunity with a client to explain the importance of regular hygiene.

Pediatric Considerations

An infant or young child should never be left unattended in a tub. Use the tub bath as an opportunity to provide an infant or child pleasant tactile stimulation.

Geriatric Considerations

Many elderly clients have alterations in mobility or balance that place them at risk of falls. An elderly person's ability to react suddenly when loss of balance is about to occur may be diminished. It may also be easy for an elderly person to get into a tub but very difficult for him to get out because of weakness in leg muscles.

Tepid Sponging

A common form of therapeutic bath is tepid sponging. The procedure promotes the controlled loss of body heat through evaporation and conduction when clients have seriously elevated fevers. Since cooling occurs slowly, temperature fluctuations are avoided. The use of tepid water prevents chilling, which can cause an elevation in body temperature from muscular shivering.

Parents of small children learn how to safely administer tepid sponge baths in the home setting. Young children are at risk of having a seizure when fevers become high. The nurse in a health care setting can begin tepid sponging while pursuing additional orders from a physician for temperature control.

Potential Nursing Diagnoses

The client with an elevated fever in need of tepid sponging may have one or more of the following nursing diagnoses:

Potential for injury related to infection

Potential fluid volume deficit related to fever and dehydration

Potential alteration in comfort related to sponging procedure

Equipment

Bath basin
Tepid water (32° C [90° F])
Bath thermometer
Washcloths

Waterproof pads
Bath blanket
Ethyl alcohol (optional)
Thermometer

Steps	Rationale
1. Wash hands.	Reduces transmission of microorganisms.
2. Explain to client that purpose of tepid sponging is to cool body slowly. Describe in brief the steps of procedure.	Procedure can be uncomfortable because of cool water application. Anxiety over procedure can increase body temperature.
3. Close room curtain or door.	Maintains client privacy.
4. Measure client's temperature and pulse.	Provides baseline to measure effects of sponging.
5. Place waterproof pads under client and remove gown.	Pads prevent soiling of bed linen. Removing gown provides access to all skin surfaces.
6. Keep bath blanket over body parts not being sponged. Close windows and door to prevent drafts in room.	Bath blanket prevents chilling.
7. Check water temperature. Add equal parts ethyl alcohol and water (optional).	Alcohol evaporates at low body temperature to increase heat loss.
8. Immerse washcloths in water and apply wet cloths under each axilla and over groin.	Axillae and groin are areas containing large superficial blood vessels. Application of sponges promotes cooler temperature of the body's core by conduction.
9. Gently sponge an extremity for 5 min. Note client's response. Opposite extremity may be covered by a cool washcloth.	Prevents sudden temperature fall and minimizes risk of developing chills.

Steps	Rationale
10. Dry extremity and reassess client's pulse and body temperature. Observe client's response to therapy.	Client's response to therapy is monitored to prevent sudden temperature change.
11. Continue sponging other extremities, back, and buttocks for 3-5 min each. Reassess temperature and pulse every 15 min.	Exposure of all body parts to sponging facilitates drop in body temperature.
12. Change water and reapply sponges to axilla and groin as needed.	Water temperature rises as result of exposure to client's warm body surface.
13. When body temperature falls to slightly above normal (38° C or 100° F), discontinue procedure.	This prevents a temperature drift to a subnormal level.
14. Dry extremities and body parts thoroughly. Cover client with a light bath blanket or sheet.	Drying and covering client prevent chilling. Excessively heavy covering may increase body temperature.
15. Dispose of equipment and change bed linen if soiled.	Controls transmission of infection.
16. Measure client's body temperature.	Indicates response to therapy.
17. Record in nurses notes time that procedure was started and terminated, vital sign changes, and client's response.	Communicates care provided in an accurate and timely fashion.

Nurse Alert

If the client begins to shiver, discontinue the procedure. Shivering causes elevation in body temperature.

Client Teaching

Teach parents of small children how to perform a tepid bath in the home. The parent should learn that a temperature above 39° C or 102° F generally indicates need for sponging.

Pediatric Considerations

A child's temperature can rise suddenly since his temperature regulation mechanisms are immature. Often the only warning sign is warm skin. It may be easier to immerse an infant or small child in a tub of tepid water than to actually sponge him. Exposure of all body parts simultaneously improves heat loss. Immersion also reduces the infants tendency to cry, which can increase body temperature. As a safety precaution the child's head and shoulders should always be firmly supported during immersion.

Geriatric Considerations

The elderly client may have altered circulatory and heat conservation mechanisms. Peripheral vasoconstriction and muscular contraction (the shivering response) do not always occur normally following a drop in the environmental temperature. During sponging it is especially important to monitor an elderly client's body temperature since a decrease can occur quickly.

Female Perineal Care

Perineal care in women involves thorough cleaning of the external genitalia. The procedure can usually be performed during the bath. Most women prefer washing their perineal areas themselves if they are physically able. Perineal care prevents and controls the spread of infection, prevents skin breakdown, promotes comfort, and maintains cleanliness.

Potential Nursing Diagnoses

Clients receiving perineal hygiene may have one or more of the following nursing diagnoses:

Potential for injury related to infection

Alteration in skin integrity related to surgical incision or episiotomy

Potential alteration in skin integrity related to incontinence or wound secretions

Knowledge deficit of basic hygiene care

Self-care deficit: bathing and hygiene

Equipment

Washbasin

Soap dish with soap

Disposable or cloth washcloths (two or three)

Bath towel

Bath blanket

Waterproof pad or bedpan

Toilet tissue

Disposable gloves

Disposable bag

Steps	Rationale
1. Explain procedure and its purpose to client.	Helps minimize anxiety during a procedure that is often embarrassing to both you and client.
2. Wash hands.	Reduces transmission of microorganisms.
3. Pull curtain around client's bed or close room door. Assemble supplies at bedside.	Maintains client's privacy.
4. Raise bed to comfortable working position.	Facilitates good body mechanics, which helps protect you from injury.
5. Lower side rail. Assist client to a dorsal recumbent position.	Provides easy access to genitalia.
6. Position waterproof pad under client's buttocks or place bedpan under client.	Prevents bedclothes from becoming wet.
7. Drape client by placing bath blanket with one corner between client's legs, one corner pointing toward each side of bed, and one corner at client's chest. Wrap bath blanket around client's far leg by bringing corner around leg and tucking it under hip. Drape near leg in same way. (Figs. 117, 118)	Prevents unnecessary exposure of body parts and maintains client's warmth and comfort during procedure.

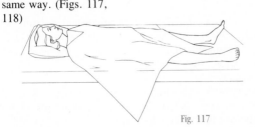

Fig. 117

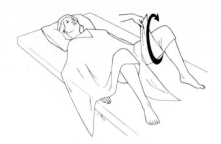

Fig. 118

Steps	Rationale
8. Raise side rail. Fill washbasin with water that is approximately 41°-43° C warm (105°-109.4° F).	Rail maintains client's safety from accidental fall. Proper water temperature prevents burns to perineum.
9. Place washbasin and toilet tissue on overbed table. Place disposable or regular washcloths in washbasin.	
10. Lower side rail and help client flex her knees and spread her legs (a client with knee or hip disease may keep her legs straight).	Provides full exposure of genitalia.
11. Put on disposable gloves. Fold lower corner of bath blanket up between client's legs onto her abdomen.	Use of gloves minimizes transmission of microorganisms. Keeping client draped until procedure begins minimizes anxiety.
12. Using your nondominant hand, retract labia from thigh. With dominant hand, wash carefully in skin folds.	Skinfolds may contain body secretions that harbor infection and cause body odor.
▪ Wipe from perineum toward anus. Repeat on opposite side using dif-	Reduces chance of transmitting microorganisms to urinary meatus.

Steps	Rationale

    ferent section of wash-
cloth. Rinse and dry
area thoroughly.

13. Separate labia with your
nondominant hand. With
other hand, wash down-
ward from pubic area to-
ward anus in one smooth
stroke. Use different section of washcloth for each
stroke. Pay particular attention to areas around labia minora, clitoris, and
vaginal orifice. (Fig. 119)

Reduces chance of transmit-
ting microorganisms to urinary
meatus.

14. If client is on a bedpan,
pour warm water over her
perineal area.

Rinsing removes soap and microorganisms more effectively
than wiping.

15. Dry perineal area thoroughly.

Retained moisture harbors microorganisms.

16. Fold center corner of bath
blanket back between
client's legs over peri-
neum. Help client off
bedpan, lower her legs,
and assist her to side-
lying position.

Bath blanket prevents unnecessary exposure of body parts.
Side-lying position provides
easy visualization of anal
area.

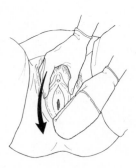

Fig. 119

Steps	Rationale
17. Clean anal area by wiping off any excess fecal material with toilet tissue. Wash area by wiping from vagina toward anus with one stroke. Discard washcloth. Repeat with clean cloth until skin is clear. (Fig. 120)	Cleaning prevents transmission of microorganisms.
18. Rinse area well and dry with towel.	Retained moisture can cause maceration of skin.
19. Remove gloves and dispose of them in proper receptacle.	Moisture and body excretions on gloves can harbor microorganisms.
20. Assist client to comfortable position and cover her with sheet.	Making client comfortable minimizes emotional stress of procedure.
21. Remove blanket and dispose of all soiled bed linen. Return unused equipment to storage area.	Reduces spread of microorganisms.
22. Raise side rail and lower bed to proper height. Return client's room to its condition before procedure.	Side rail protects client from fall. Clean environment promotes client's comfort.

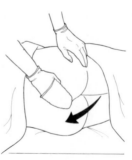

Fig. 120

Steps	Rationale
23. Wash your hands.	Reduces transmission of microorganisms.
24. Record in nurse's notes and report any observations (e.g., amount and character of discharge, condition of genitalia).	Timely recording ensures accurate documentation of care.

Nurse Alert

The presence of foul-smelling discharge may indicate an infection and require a physician's attention.

Client Teaching

Adolescent girls should learn basic perineal hygiene and understand why they are predisposed to urinary tract infections.

Pediatric Considerations

A common problem among infants is diaper rash, created by the hot humid environment under the diaper. Airing and cooling are the most effective ways to promote healing. Change diapers as soon as they become wet. Remove excess clothing and occlusive diaper coverings.

Geriatric Considerations

Elderly women commonly have atrophy of the external genitalia along with a reduction in hair growth over the perineum.

Male Perineal Care

A male client requires special attention during perineal care, especially if he is uncircumcised. The foreskin causes secretions to accumulate easily around the crown of the penis near the urethral meatus. Penile cancer occurs more frequently in uncircumcised males and is believed to be related to cleanliness. Bacteria that collect under the foreskin act on desquamated cells to produce smegma, a substance irritating to the glans penis and prepuce.

As is the case with female perineal care, the male client requires hygiene not only as a routine part of the bath but also whenever urinary incontinence occurs and as a part of Foley catheter care.

Potential Nursing Diagnoses

A male client in need of perineal hygiene may have one or more of the following nursing diagnoses:

Potential for injury related to skin infection

Potential impairment in skin integrity related to incontinence or accumulated secretions

Knowledge deficit regarding basic hygiene care

Self-care deficit: bathing and hygiene

Equipment

Washbasin	Bath blanket
Soap dish with soap	Waterproof pad or bedpan
Disposable or cloth washcloths (two or three)	Toilet tissue
	Disposable gloves
Bath towel	Disposable bag

Steps	Rationale
1. Explain procedure and its purpose to client.	Helps minimize anxiety during a procedure that is often embarrassing to both you and client.
2. Wash hands.	Reduces transmission of microorganisms.
3. Pull curtain around client's bed or close room door. Assemble supplies at the bedside.	Maintains client privacy.
4. Raise bed to comfortable working position.	Facilitates good body mechanics and safety.
5. Lower side rail. Assist client to a supine position.	Provides easy access to genitalia.
6. Position waterproof pad under client's buttocks or place bedpan under client.	Prevents bedclothes from becoming wet.
7. Drape client by placing bath blanket with one corner between his legs, a corner pointing toward each side of body, and a corner over his chest.	Prevents unnecessary exposure before beginning procedure.
8. Raise side rail. Fill washbasin with water that is approximately 41°-43° C (105°-109.4° F).	Rail maintains client's safety. Proper water temperature prevents burns to perineum.
9. Place washbasin and toilet tissue on overbed table. Place disposable or regular washcloths in washbasin.	Equipment placed within your reach prevents accidental spills.
10. Lower top corner of bath blanket below client's perineum. Gently raise penis and place bath towel underneath it.	Towel prevents moisture from collecting in inguinal area.

Steps	Rationale
11. Gently grasp shaft of penis. If client is uncircumcised, retract foreskin.	Secretions capable of harboring microorganisms collect underneath foreskin.
12. Wash the tip of penis at urethral meatus first. Using a circular motion, clean from meatus outward. Do not allow soap to get into meatus. Discard washcloth and repeat until penis is clean. Rinse and dry gently. (Fig. 121)	Cleaning moves from area of least contamination to most contaminated preventing entrance of microorganisms into urethra.
13. Return foreskin to its natural position.	Tightening of foreskin around shaft of penis can cause localized edema and discomfort.
14. Wash shaft of penis with gentle but firm downward strokes. Pay special attention to underlying surface of penis.	Vigorous massage of penis can lead to erection, which can cause embarassment for client.
15. Rinse and dry penis thoroughly. Instruct client to spread his legs apart slightly.	Spreading legs provides easy access to scrotal tissues.

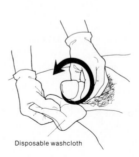

Disposable washcloth

Fig. 121

Steps	Rationale
16. Gently clean scrotum. Lift testicles carefully and wash underlying skin-folds. Rinse and dry.	Pressure on scrotal tissues can be very painful to client.
17. Fold bath blanket back over client's perineum and assist client in turning to a side-lying position.	Bath blanket maintains client's comfort and minimizes anxiety during procedure. Side-lying position provides access to anal area.
18. Clean anal area by wiping off any excess fecal material with toilet tissue. Wash area by wiping from perineum toward anus with one stroke. Discard washcloth. Repeat with a clean cloth until skin is clear.	Prevents transmission of microorganisms.
19. Rinse area well and dry with towel.	Retained moisture can promote skin breakdown.
20. Remove gloves and dispose of them in proper receptable.	Moisture and body excretions on gloves can harbor microorganisms.
21. Assist client to a comfortable position and cover him with sheet.	Making client comfortable minimizes emotional stress of procedure.
22. Raise side rail and lower bed to proper height. Return client's room to its condition before procedure.	Side rail protects client from falling. Clean environment promotes client comfort.
23. Remove blanket and dispose of all soiled bed linen. Return unused equipment to storage area.	Reduces transfer of microorganisms.
24. Wash hands.	Reduces transmission of microorganisms.

Steps	Rationale
25. Record procedure in nurse's notes and report any observations (e.g., amount and character of discharge, condition of genitalia.)	Timely recording ensures accurate documentation of care.

Nurse Alert

If a male client has an erection due to manipulation of the shaft of the penis, simply defer the procedure until later to avoid embarassing him. In the presence of any ulcers, lesions, or discharge, wear disposable gloves. These may be indicative of venereal disease. Thorough rinsing is necessary to remove soap, which can be very irritating to the urinary meatus.

Client Teaching

During perineal care the nurse can instruct the young male client on testicular self-examinations. Testicular cancer is the most common form of solid tumor in males between ages of 15 and 35.

Pediatric Considerations

In an infant the prepuce is normally tight for the first several months and should not be retracted for cleaning. Accidental tearing of the membranes may occur.

Geriatric Considerations

In elderly clients the testes diminish in size. This is a normal process of aging.

Administering a Backrub

The nurse may offer to rub a client's back during the course of bathing or when it is advantageous to help a client relax. A backrub or massage is a useful pain relief measure. It eases muscular tension, stimulates circulation to the skin, and helps a person relax. Normally the nurse should take at least 3 to 5 minutes to give a thorough backrub.

Potential Nursing Diagnoses

Clients who receive a backrub may have any of the following nursing diagnoses:

Alteration in comfort related to musculoskeletal or incisional pain

Anxiety related to fear of unknown or grieving

Potential impairment in skin integrity related to pressure sites and drying

Equipment

Bath blanket
Bath towel
Lotion (cream, alcohol, or powder)

Steps	Rationale
1. Explain procedure and desired position to client.	Helps relieve anxiety about procedure.
2. Adjust bed to a high comfortable position.	Reduces strain on your back.

Steps	Rationale
4. Expose client's back, shoulders, upper arms, and buttocks. Cover rest of body with bath blanket. Lay a towel alongside client's back.	Body parts should not be exposed unnecessarily.
5. Wash your hands in warm water. Warm lotion either in your hands or by placing container under warm water.	Cold causes muscle tension.
6. Explain to client that lotion may feel cold and wet.	Warning client reduces startle response.
7. Apply lotion to sacral area and stroke upward from buttocks to shoulders, over upper arms, and back to buttocks, using a continuous firm stroke. Follow muscle groups. Do not let your hands leave client's skin. Continue for at least 3 min. (Fig. 122)	Continuous contact is soothing and stimulates circulation to tissues.

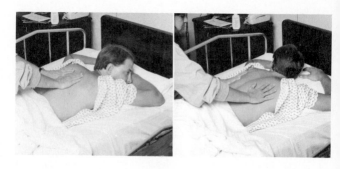

Fig. 122

Steps	Rationale
8. Knead skin by grasping tissue between your thumb and fingers. Knead upward along one side of spine from buttock to shoulder and nape of the neck. Knead or stroke down. Repeat along other side of spine. (Fig. 123)	Increases circulation to muscles. Continuous motion is soothing and relieves muscle tension.
9. End massage with long stroking movements and tell client you are ending it.	Long stroking is most soothing massage movement.
10. Wipe excess lubricant from client's back with bath towel. Retie gown or assist with pajamas. Help client to comfortable position.	Excess lotion can be an irritant. Comfortable position enhances backrub's effects.
11. Dispose of soiled towel and wash your hands.	Promotes infection control.
12. Record in nurse's notes client's response and condition of skin.	Documents therapy in timely manner.

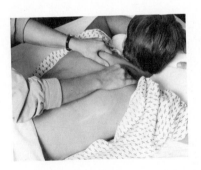

Fig. 123

Nurse Alert

Avoid direct massage over any areas of abrasion. A client with a history of cardiac irregularities should be watched closely for changes in heart rate during the procedure. Gentle massage may increase the heart rate and systolic blood pressure.

Client Teaching

Discuss with the client the benefits of back massage and relaxation exercises as measures to ease tension.

Pediatric Considerations

Infants or children do not require a complete backrub. However, tactile stimulation of the skin can be very pleasurable to them.

Geriatric Considerations

Use extra caution in monitoring the vital signs of elderly clients, who may be at risk of alterations in heart rate. Also apply gentle massage, since an elderly person's skin is often thin and fragile.

Decubitus Ulcer Care

The best treatment for decubitus ulcers is prevention. Keeping clients mobile, maintaining optimal nutrition, and providing good skin care are a few of the ways to keep pressure sores from developing. When clients become immobilized, there are a variety of pressure-relieving mattresses and beds that can also assist in preventing decubiti.

Once a bedsore develops, there may be a need for additional therapy. The use of topical agents on decubitus ulcers is quick and easy. No single topical agent, however, has been found to be most effective. The choice of agents depends on the depth of the ulcer.

Potential Nursing Diagnoses

Clients in need of topical applications for decubitus ulcer care may have any of the following nursing diagnoses:

Actual impairment of skin integrity related to decubiti
Sensory alteration related to reduced tactile stimulation
Impaired physical mobility
Alteration in peripheral tissue perfusion

Equipment

Washbasin, warm water, soap, washcloth, bath towel
Normal saline or hydrogen peroxide in sterile cup
Prescribed topical agent:

Enzymes: collagenase, fibrinolysin, deoxyribonuclease, or sutilains
Antiseptics: povidone-iodine, ointment or solution; merbromin, 5% or 10% solution; sodium hypochlorite, 1:12 or 1:20 solution

Oxydizing agents: benzoyl peroxide, 20%; hydrogen peroxide, half strength
Dextranomer beads (Debrisan)
Sterile gauze dressing
Hypoallergenic tape
Disposable or sterile gloves
Protective paste such as zinc oxide (optional)

Steps	Rationale
1. Wash hands	Reduces transmission of infection.
2. Close room door or bedside curtains.	Maintains client's privacy.
3. Position client comfortably with area of decubitus ulcer and surrounding skin easily accessible.	Area should be accessible for cleaning of ulcer and surrounding skin.
4. Assemble needed supplies at bedside. Open sterile packages and topical solution containers.	Sterile supplies should be ready for easy application so you can use sterile gloves without contaminating them.
5. Remove bed linen and client's gown to expose ulcer and surrounding skin. Keep remaining body parts draped.	Prevents unnecessary exposure of body parts.
6. Explain to client that you are going to clean decubitus ulcer and apply medication over its surface. Warn client that he may feel sensation of burning or coolness.	Preparatory explanations relieve client's anxiety and promote cooperation during procedure.
7. Wash skin surrounding ulcer gently with warm water and soap.	Cleaning skin surface reduces number of resident bacteria.
8. Rinse area thoroughly with water.	Soap can be irritating to skin.

Steps	Rationale
9. Gently dry skin thoroughly by patting lightly with towel.	Retained moisture causes maceration of skin layers. Rubbing with towel may injure sensitive tissues.
10. Apply enzymes:	
▪ Don sterile gloves (Skill 5-6).	Aseptic technique must be maintained while cleaning ulcer and applying topical agent.
▪ Clean ulcer thoroughly with normal saline or hydrogen peroxide on moistened sterile gauze dressing.	Removes ointment and digested material. Previously applied enzymes may require soaking for removal.
▪ Keeping gloves sterile, place small amount of enzyme ointment in palm of hand.	It is not necessary to apply thick layer of ointment. Thin layer absorbs and acts more effectively. Excess medication can irritate surrounding skin.
▪ Soften medication by rubbing briskly in palm of hand.	Makes ointment easier to apply to ulcer.
▪ Apply a thin even layer of ointment over ulcer. Do not apply enzyme to surrounding skin.	Proper distribution of ointment ensures effective action. Enzyme can cause burning, paresthesia, and dermatitis to surrounding skin.
▪ Moisten gauze dressing in saline and apply directly over ulcer.	Protects wound. Keeping ulcer surface moist reduces time needed for healing. Skin cells normally live in moist environment.
▪ Cover moistened gauze with single dry gauze and tape securely in place.	Prevents bacteria from entering moist dressing.
11. Apply antiseptic:	
a. Superficial ulcers	
▪ Don sterile gloves (Skill 5-6).	Maintains aseptic technique.

Steps	Rationale
▪ Moisten sterile gauze in normal saline and gently clean ulcer surface.	Removes wound exudate and any remaining antiseptic containing bacteria.
▪ Moisten sterile gauze with antiseptic solution and paint surface of ulcer.	Distributes antiseptic over entire area to effectively reduce bacterial growth.
▪ Leave ulcer open to air.	If superficial epidermal skin layer is only layer affected, keeping wound dry promotes better healing.
b. Deep ulcers	
▪ Don sterile gloves (Skill 5-6).	Maintains aseptic technique.
▪ Moisten sterile gauze with antiseptic solution and gently clean ulcer surface.	Reduces number of pathogenic organisms on wound surface.
▪ Moisten sterile gauze with normal saline and rinse ulcer thoroughly.	Antiseptic solution left remaining on deeper tissue layers may cause irritation.
▪ If gloves become soiled remove and reapply new pair.	Prevents contaminating clean ulcer surface.
▪ Apply antiseptic ointment to dominant gloved hand and spread ointment in and around ulcer.	Antiseptic ointment causes minimal tissue irritation. All surfaces of wound must be covered to effectively control bacterial growth.
▪ Apply sterile gauze pad over ulcer and tape securely in place.	Protects ulcer and prevents removal of ointment during turning or repositioning.
12. Apply oxidizing agent:	
▪ Don sterile gloves (Skill 5-6).	Maintains aseptic technique.

Steps	Rationale
▪ Moisten gauze in saline and clean ulcer surface gently.	Removes any wound exudate.
▪ Spread zinc oxide paste over skin surface surrounding ulcer.	Oxidizing agents can be caustic to normal tissues.
▪ Apply single layer of gauze dressing moistened in oxidizing solution over the ulcer (do not apply full-strength peroxide).	Coats wound surface and retains exposure to tissue surface.
▪ Apply dry gauze dressing over ulcer.	Protects ulcer and prevents loosening or pulling away of moist dressing.
13. Apply dextranomer beads:	
▪ Don disposable gloves (Skill 5-6).	Beads usually applied to deeper wounds that are already infected. Gloves reduce contact with infectious material.
▪ Soak ulcer in normal saline by applying moist gauze to ulcer. Allow gauze to remain in place for several minutes.	Soaking removes dried beads that adhere to skin.
▪ Hold container of beads approximately 2.5 cm (1 inch) above ulcer site and lightly sprinkle 5 mm diameter layer over wound.	Layer of insoluble powder is needed to absorb wound exudate.
▪ Apply gauze dressing over ulcer.	Holds beads in place and protects wound.
14. Reposition client comfortably off decubitus ulcer.	Avoids accidental removal of dressings.
15. Remove gloves and dispose of soiled supplies. Wash hands.	Reduces transmission of microorganisms.

Steps	Rationale
16. Record in nurse's notes appearance of ulcer. Describe type of topical agent used, dressing applied, and client's response.	Baseline observations coupled with subsequent inspections reveal progress of healing. Documents care provided.
17. Report any worsening of ulcer's appearance to nurse in charge or physician.	May indicate need for additional therapy.

Nurse Alert

Do not use a tongue blade to apply ointment. The blade is not sterile, and it can cause too much pressure against sensitive tissues. If necrotic tissue is present, a physician may be needed to surgically debride the ulcer.

Client Teaching

Explain the importance of regular turning and proper nutrition for treatment and prevention of ulcers. This may improve the client's cooperation with preventive care.

Pediatric Considerations

Pressure sores rarely develop in children, except in those with serious nutritional deficits.

Geriatric Considerations

The skin of elderly clients is less elastic and more dry than that of younger clients, and the tissue mass is reduced. Often elderly persons have low serum protein levels. Use tape with caution since brusque removal can cause skin burns or tears.

Nail and Foot Care

The nurse provides routine nail and foot care to prevent infection, foot odors, and injury to soft tissue. Often a client is unaware of a foot or toenail problem until pain or discomfort develops. The integrity of the feet and toenails is important to maintaining normal function of the feet so a person can stand and walk comfortably. The most common fingernail, foot, and toenail problems result from abuse or poor care such as biting nails or trimming them improperly, exposure to harsh chemicals, and wearing ill-fitting shoes. Disease, poor nutrition, and the physiological processes of aging also impair integrity of the nails.

Potential Nursing Diagnoses

Clients who receive nail and foot care may have a variety of nursing diagnoses depending on the condition of the feet and nails and the disease processes contributing to any alterations:

Impairment in skin integrity related to calluses and/or corns

Alteration in comfort related to foot and/or nail disorders

Reduced tissue perfusion related to arterial insufficiency

Altered mobility related to foot discomfort

Knowledge deficit regarding nail and foot care

Equipment

Washbasin	Emery board or nail file
Bath towel, face towel	Lotion
Washcloth	Disposable bath mats
Emesis basin	Paper towels
Nail clippers, orange stick	Disposable gloves

Steps	Rationale
1. Explain procedure to client.	Promotes clients participation in care procedures.
2. Obtain physician's order if agency policy requires it.	During cutting, client's skin may accidentally be broken. Certain clients are more at risk of infection.
3. Arrange equipment on overbed table. Pull curtain around bed or close room door.	Easy access to equipment prevents delays. Maintaining client's privacy reduces anxiety.
4. Assist client to bedside chair if possible. Place disposable bath mat on floor under client's feet. Place call light within client's reach.	Chair makes it easier for client to immerse feet in basin. Call light within reach assures his safety.
5. Fill washbasin with water at 43°-44° C (109°-110° F).	Warm water softens nails, reduces inflammation of skin, and promotes circulation.
6. Place basin on bath mat and help client place his feet in basin.	
7. Adjust overbed table to low position and place it over client's lap.	Easy access prevents accidental spills.
8. Fill emesis basin with water at 43°-44° C (109°-110° F) and place on paper towel on overbed table.	Warm water softens nails and thickened epidermal cells.
9. Instruct client to place his fingers in basin with his arms in a comfortable position.	Allows client to retain position.
10. Allow client's toenails and fingernails to soak for 10-20 minutes. Rewarm water in 10 min.	Softening of cuticles promotes easy removal of dead cells.

Steps	Rationale
11. Clean gently under finger-nails with orange stick. Remove emesis basin and dry fingers thoroughly.	Orange stick can be used to remove debris that harbors microorganisms. Thorough drying impedes fungal growth and prevents maceration of tissues.
12. With nail clippers, clip fingernails straight across and even with tops of fingers. Shape nails with an emery board or nail file. (Fig. 124)	Cutting straight across prevents splitting of nail margins and formation of sharp nail spikes that can irritate lateral nail margins. Filing prevents cutting nail too close to nail bed.
13. Push the cuticle back gently with orange stick.	Reduces incidence of inflamed cuticles.
14. Move overbed table away from client.	
15. Put on disposable gloves and scrub callused areas of client's feet with wash-cloth.	Gloves prevent transmission of fungal infections to you. Friction removes dead skin layers.
16. Clean gently under client's toenails with orange stick. Remove feet from basin and dry them thoroughly.	Removal of debris and excess moisture reduces chances of infection.

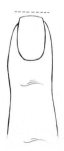

Fig. 124

Steps	Rationale
17. Clean and trim toenails using procedures in Steps 11 and 12.	
18. Apply lotion to client's feet and then assist him back to bed and into a comfortable position.	Lotion lubricates dry skin by helping to retain moisture.
19. Make sure that call light is within reach. Raise side rail.	Call light and side rail provide for client safety.
20. Clean and return equipment and supplies to proper place. Dispose of soiled linen. Wash your hands.	Controls transmission of microorganisms
21. Record procedure in nurse's notes and report any pertinent observations (e.g., breaks in skin or areas of inflammation).	Accurate documentation is timely and descriptive.

Nurse Alert

Clients with diabetes may have peripheral neuropathies causing reduced sensation. Therefore, test the water temperature carefully. Take extra care in trimming the nails of clients with diabetes mellitus or peripheral vascular disease. These clients tend to have poor wound healing capabilities and a slight cut could lead to serious infection.

Client Teaching

During nail care, instruct the client on proper techniques so routine care can be performed at home. Educate the client about safe use of home remedies for foot and nail care. Moleskin should be used to protect areas of the feet with corns or calluses. The moleskin does not cause local pressure as corn pads do. Chemical preparations used to remove corns can cause burns and ulcerations. Clients should be warned against cutting off corns or calluses since the risk of infection is great. Wrapping lamb's wool around toes can effectively reduce irritation to the skin.

Clients should also be taught about proper footwear. Socks can be worn to absorb perspiration. Footwear must always be clean to avoid infection. Women should be advised against wearing tight nylons or garters, which can constrict circulation. A person's shoes must not fit too tightly. It is recommended that a ¾-inch space between the great toe and the widest part of the shoe be present when a person stands. Clients should not try to cut hardened or hypertrophied nails. Referral to a podiatrist is a safer measure.

Pediatric Considerations

Infants and young children require routine trimming of fingernails and toenails to prevent cuts in the skin. Soaking is usually unnecessary. A child with short ragged fingernails may be a habitual nail biter. The presence of uncut nails with dirt accumulated under the edges is a sign of poor hygiene practices.

Geriatric Considerations

Elderly clients are more likely to have foot or toenail problems since poor vision, uncoordination, obesity, or inability to bend over can impede their performance of proper care. It is common for an elderly person to have dry feet and fissures of the feet and toes due to reduced sebaceous gland secretion and dehydration of tissue cells. The elderly also are more likely to suffer from conditions such as diabetes, heart or renal failure, and cerebrovascular accidents, all of which can contribute to foot and nail problems.

Care of Contact

Lenses

Contact lens care is important to maintaining a client's optimal visual acuity and preventing corneal irritation or infection. Clients generally prefer to care for their own lenses when possible. However, illness may necessitate the nurse's assistance. Contact lens care includes cleaning, proper application and removal, and storage. Clients usually have a preferred method of caring for their lenses. When it becomes necessary for the nurse to assist with lens care, the client's preferences should be considered.

Potential Nursing Diagnoses

Clients receiving contact lens care may have any of the following nursing diagnoses:

Alteration in comfort related to corneal irritation

Alteration in sensory perception related to visual alterations

Self-care deficit: hygiene, related to physical restrictions

Equipment

Contact lenses
Contact lens storage case
Sterile saline
Bath towel
Lens cleaner (optional)
Wetting solution

Steps	Rationale
1. Discuss procedure with client.	Client can assist in planning by explaining technique that he feels may aid in removal and insertion. He may be anxious as you retract his eyelids and manipulate contact lens. Therefore be especially gentle.
2. Have client assume a supine or sitting position in bed or chair.	Provides easy access for you to retract eyelids and manipulate contact lens.
3. Wash hands.	Reduces transmission of microorganisms.
4. Place towel just below client's face.	Catches lens if one should accidentally fall from the eye.

Removal of Soft Lenses

1. Add a few drops of sterile saline to client's eye.	Lubricates eye to facilitate lens removal
2. Ask client to look forward.	Eases tipping of lens during removal.
3. Using thumb, retract lower eyelid.	Exposes lower edge of lens.
4. With pad of index finger of same hand, slide lens off cornea onto white of eye.	Positions lens for easy grasping. Use of finger pad prevents injury to cornea and damage to lens.
5. Place upper eyelid down gently with thumb of other hand and compress lens slightly between thumb and index finger.	Causes soft lens to double up. Air enters underneath lens to release suction.
6. Grasp lens and lift out. Hold lens in cupped hand.	Protects lens from damage.
7. Place lens in proper cup of storage case. Be sure that it is centered properly.	Ensures that proper lens will be reinserted into correct eye.
8. Repeat Steps 1 through 7 for other lens. Secure cover over storage case.	Proper storage prevents cracking or tearing.

Steps	Rationale
9. Dispose of towel and wash hands.	Reduces transmission of infection.

Removal of Hard Lenses

Steps	Rationale
1. Be sure that lens is positioned directly over cornea. If it is not, apply gentle pressure against lower eyelid with thumb or index finger and position lens properly	Correct position of lens allows for easy removal from eye.
2. Place index finger on outer corner of client's eye and draw skin gently back toward his ear.	Tightens lids against eyeball.
3. Instruct client to blink.	Should cause lens to dislodge and pop out.
4. If lens fails to pop out, carefully retract eyelid beyond edges of lens.	Pressure causes upper edge of lens to tip forward.
5. Allow both eyelids to close slightly and grasp lens as it rises from eye.	Causes lens to slide off easily
6. Cup lens in your hand.	Protects lens from breakage.
7. Place lens in proper cup labeled *L* for left eye or *R* for right eye. Center lens in cup.	Both lenses may not have same prescription. Proper storage prevents cracking, tearing, or chipping.
8. Repeat Steps 1 through 7 for other lens. Secure cover over storage case.	Proper storage prevents damage to lens.
9. Dispose of towel and wash hands.	Controls spread of infection and keeps client's environment neat.

Cleaning of Lenses (Both Soft and Hard)

Steps	Rationale
1. Wash hands	Reduces transmission of microorganisms

Steps	Rationale
2. Assemble supplies at bedside.	Provides easy access to supplies
3. Open lens container carefully. Do not flip lens caps open suddenly.	Prevents lenses from being accidentally spilled or flipped out of case.
4. If lens has been soaking in disinfectant overnight, simply rinse with either saline (soft lenses) or tap water (hard lenses). Rinse thoroughly.	Special disinfecting solutions can effectively clean lenses soaked over 4 hours.
5. If lenses have not been disinfected, pick them up one at a time by your fingertips and apply lens cleaner to both sides.	It is easier to manipulate and clean lenses using fingertips.
6. Spread lens cleaner evenly over lens surface, using your fingertips or cotton ball or applicator. Hold close over bath towel.	Cleans all surfaces for microorganisms.
7. After cleaning, pour warm tap water over lens while holding it over emesis basin. Gently rub lens surface during rinsing.	Removes debris from lens surface.
8. Reinsert lens immediately after cleaning.	Prevents contamination due to placing of lens in storage container.

Insertion of Soft Lenses

1. Place right lens concave side up, like a bowl, on tip of index finger of your dominant hand.	Inner surface of lens should face up so it is applied against cornea.
2. Have client look up or to side. Retract both his eyelids.	Soft lenses do not adhere as easily as hard lenses. Client's position eases application to surface of eye. Lens should fit easily between eyelid margins.

Steps	Rationale
3. Place soft lens directly over sclera. It may be necessary to press lightly to make lens adhere to eye.	Will allow lens to move over cornea.
4. Have client close his eye and roll it toward lens.	Centers soft lens over cornea.
5. Be sure that lens is centered properly by asking client if his vision is blurred.	If lens slips to side of cornea or into conjunctival sac, vision will blur.
6. If client's vision is blurred: ■ Retract his eyelids and locate position of lens. ■ Ask client to look in opposite direction from lens and with your index finger, apply pressure to lower eyelid margin. Position lens over cornea. ■ Have client look slowly toward lens.	Repositions lens over center of cornea as client looks toward lens.
7. Repeat Steps 1 through 6 for other eye.	
8. Assist client to comfortable position.	Promotes client comfort.
9. Wash your hands and discard soiled supplies. Store lens container and wetting and cleaning solutions in client's bedside drawer.	Prevents infection and maintains a neat environment.

Insertion of Hard Lenses

1. Place right lens concave side up on tip of index finger of your dominant hand. (Fig. 125)	Ensures easy insertion. Inner surface of lens should face up so it is applied against cornea.
2. Apply drop of wetting solution to inside of lens surface.	Lubricates lens so it slides easily over and adheres to cornea.

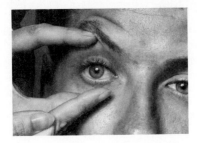

Fig. 125

Steps	Rationale
3. While retracting client's upper and lower eyelids, instruct him to look straight ahead. Place lens gently over center of cornea.	Hard lens is rigid and can be placed as client looks straight ahead. Retraction of lids promotes easy insertion between lid margins.
4. Ask client to close his eyes briefly and avoid blinking.	Helps to secure position of lens.
5. Be sure that lens is centered properly by asking client if his vision is blurred.	If lens slips to side of cornea or into conjunctival sac, vision will blur.
6. Repeat Steps 1 through 5 for left eye.	
7. Assist client to comfortable position.	Promotes client comfort.
8. Wash your hands and discard soiled supplies. Store lens container and wetting and cleaning solutions in client's bedside drawer.	Prevents infection and maintains a neat environment.

Nurse Alert

A critically ill client admitted to hospital should be assessed for the presence of contact lenses. If they are present but not detected, they can cause serious corneal injury. Suction cups are available to lift a contact lens off the cornea.

Client Teaching

Clients who are relatively new wearers of contact lenses should be instructed in all aspects of lens care. Information to emphasize includes duration that lenses can safely remain inserted, cleaning methods, signs of corneal irritation, insertion techniques, and situations in which lenses should not be worn.

Pediatric Considerations

Parents or older children should learn all aspects of contact lens care.

Geriatric Considerations

Elderly clients who are able to wear contact lenses should be carefully assessed for their ability to insert and remove a lens. Any hand tremors or impairment in fine motor coordination or ability to grasp small objects may prevent them from performing self-care. If an older client suddenly becomes ill, a family member or friend should know how to remove contact lenses.

Care of Hearing Aids

A hearing aid intensifies the sound reaching the tympanic membrane (eardrum). Each client requires a different level of sound amplification. The aid consists of an ear mold, a battery compartment, a microphone and amplifier, and a connecting tube. The "behind-the-ear" device is the most common type used. (Fig. 126)

Care of a hearing aid includes proper cleaning, battery care, and storage. The nurse must also know the correct way to insert a hearing aid for a dependent client.

Potential Nursing Diagnoses

The client who requires a hearing aid may have either or both of the following nursing diagnoses:

Sensory alteration related to hearing impairment

Knowledge deficit related to care of a hearing aid

Equipment

Emesis basin
Mild soap and water
Pipe cleaner (optional)
Syringe needle (optional)
Soft towel
Washcloth
Storage case

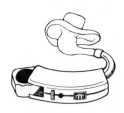

Fig. 126

Steps	Rationale
1. Wash hands.	Reduces transfer of microorganisms.
2. Assemble supplies at bedside table or sink area.	Prevents delays in procedure.
3. Remove hearing aid from client's ear.	Eliminates unpleasant feedback squeal (harsh whistling sound), which can be caused by proximity of the aid to objects near wearer's body.
4. Determine if new battery is needed. ▪ Close "battery door." ▪ Turn volume slowly to high. ▪ Cup hand over ear mold. ▪ If no sound, replace battery and check again.	Batteries usually need replacing after 1 week of daily wear.
5. Check that plastic connecting tube is not twisted or cracked.	Cracked or twisted tube prevents transmission of sound.
6. Check to see if ear mold is cracked or has rough edges.	Can cause irritation to external ear canal.
7. Check for accumulation of cerumen around ear mold and plugging of bore (opening) in mold.	Prevents clear sound reception and transmission.

Cleaning

1. Detach ear mold from hearing aid.	Moisture entering battery and transmitter will cause permanent damage.
2. Add warm water and soap to emesis basin. Soak ear mold for few minutes. Be careful not to soak too long since cement holding ear mold to aid can become softened.	Removes cerumen that can accumulate on mold.

Steps	Rationale
3. Wash client's ear canal with washcloth moistened in soap and water. Rinse and dry.	Removes cerumen and debris.
4. If cerumen has built up in bore of ear mold, carefully clean hole with tip of syringe needle.	Wax will prevent normal sound transmission.
5. Rinse ear mold in clear water.	Soap may form residue that blocks opening in mold.
6. Allow mold to dry thoroughly after wiping with a soft towel.	Water droplets left in connecting tube could enter hearing aid and damage parts.
7. (optional) Clean connecting tube carefully with pipe cleaner.	Removes moisture and debris, which can interfere with sound transmission and hearing aid function.
8. Reconnect ear mold to hearing aid.	Reassemble before inserting or storing hearing aid.

Storage

1. Open "battery door."	Ensures that there will be no contact, which would cause battery to run down.

2. Store hearing aid in storage case if client is about to do any of following:
    Bathe
    Walk in rain
    Use a hair dryer
    Sit in sun or under heat lamp
    Go to surgery or major diagnostic procedure
    Sleep
Or is diaphoretic
	Protects against damage and breakage.

Steps	Rationale

Insertion

1. To reinsert hearing aid, first check battery and replace as needed.

   Ensures proper sound amplification.

2. Turn aid off and turn volume control down.

   Protects client from sudden exposure to sound.

3. Place ear mold in external auditory meatus (ear canal). Be sure that ear bore in mold is first placed in ear canal. Shape of mold indicates which is correct ear. Slowly and with care, twist mold until it feels snug.

   Proper fit ensures optimal sound transmission.

4. Gently bring connecting tube up and over ear toward back. Avoid kinking. Hearing aid fits around the upper ear.

   Ensures correct function of hearing aid device and maintains client comfort.

5. Adjust volume gradually to comfortable level for talking to client in regular voice at a distance of 1-1.25 meters (3-4 feet).

   Gradual adjustment prevents exposing client to harsh squeal or feedback. Client should hear you comfortably.

6. Remove soiled equipment from bedside and dispose of used supplies. Wash your hands.

   Maintains clean environment and reduces risk of infection.

7. If client is going to surgery or other special procedure, record removal and storage in nurse's notes.

   Protects you from liability if aid is lost.

Client Teaching

Discuss with the client guidelines for hearing aid use and tips for care: avoiding exposure to excess heat or cold, not dropping the aid on a hard surface, changing the battery over a towel or bed, not exposing the aid to moisture, not applying hair spray while wearing the aid, cleaning the battery to remove corrosion. The battery should be stored in a cool dry place. Keep the contacts clean by removing residue with a pencil eraser. Remove the battery when the aid is being stored.

Pediatric Considerations

A hearing deficit in children can cause serious developmental problems, including speech impediments, poor recognition of verbal cues, delayed socialization, and impaired learning.

Geriatric Considerations

Isolation and social withdrawal are common among persons with a hearing deficit. Often the elderly client is sensitive about admitting that he cannot hear clearly. The nurse should use good communication techniques to help the person understand what is being said.

Brushing Teeth of a Dependent Client

It is frequently necessary for the nurse to assist a client when illness prevents him from being able to perform routine dental hygiene. Clients restricted from eating or drinking as a result of therapy, illness, or reduced consciousness have thick foul-tasting secretions that develop within their mouths. Certain conditions imposed by illness or resulting from therapies can cause a client's oral cavity to become excessively dry or irritated. Often a dependent client will have tubes or an airway exiting from his mouth that add to his discomfort. Assisting the client with regular brushing provides an intact well hydrated mucosa, clean tooth surfaces, and a sense of comfort. The frequency of care should be based upon the condition of the oral cavity and the client's level of comfort.

Potential Nursing Diagnoses

Clients requiring assistance with toothbrushing may have any of the following nursing diagnoses:

Impaired mucous membrane integrity related to dehydration and local irritation of airway

Alteration in comfort related to pain within oral cavity

Altered nutritional intake related to oral pain

Self-care deficit: oral hygiene, related to physical restrictions

Knowledge deficit regarding oral hygiene

Equipment

Toothbrush with straight handle and small soft bristles
Toothpaste or dentifrice
Water glass with cool water
Mouthwash (optional)
Straw
Emesis basin
Face towel and paper towels

Steps	Rationale
1. Explain procedure to client and inquire about his preferences regarding hygiene aids.	Certain clients may feel uncomfortable about having you care for their basic hygiene needs. Participation by client will promote his relaxation during procedure.
2. Wash hands.	Reduces transmission of microorganisms.
3. Place paper towels on overbed table and arrange other equipment within easy reach.	Towels collect spills from emesis basin.
4. Pull curtain or close room door.	Provides privacy.
5. Raise bed to a comfortable working position. Raise head of bed to position in which client is comfortable. Move or help client move to a position near you.	Raising bed prevents muscle strain as you attend to client's needs. Semi-Fowler position prevents client from aspirating or choking.
6. Lower side rail and place towel on client's chest.	Prevents soiling of bed linen.
7. Position overbed table within easy reach and adjust height as needed.	Ensures smooth procedure.

Steps	Rationale
8. Apply toothpaste to tooth-brush and hold toothbrush over emesis basin. Pour a small amount of water over end of brush.	Moisture aids in distribution of toothpaste over tooth surfaces.
9. Brush inner and outer surfaces of upper and lower teeth, always brushing from gum onto crown of each tooth. Apply brush at a 45-degree angle to gum line and use short strokes. (Fig. 127) Brush one tooth at a time. Clean biting surfaces of teeth by holding brush parallel to teeth and brushing gently back and forth. Brush sides of teeth also by moving bristles back and forth.	45-degree angle allows bristles to clean under gum line, where most plaque and tartar accumulate. Back-and-forth motion dislodges food particles caught between teeth and along chewing surfaces.
10. Hold brush at 45-degree angle and lightly brush over surface and sides of tongue. Avoid initiating gag reflex.	Microorganisms grow abundantly on tongue's surface. Gagging causes discomfort and may result in aspiration of toothpaste.
11. Allow client to rinse his mouth thoroughly by taking several sips of water, swishing it across all tooth surfaces, and spitting it into emesis basin.	Removes food particles.

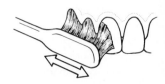

Fig. 127

Steps	Rationale
12. Allow client to gargle or rinse his mouth with mouthwash.	Leaves a pleasant taste in mouth.
13. Assist client to a comfortable position, remove bedside table, raise side rail, and lower bed to its original position.	Provides client's comfort and safety.
14. Wipe off overbed table, discard soiled linen and paper towels in appropriate container, and return equipment to proper place.	Controls transmission of microorganisms.
15. Wash your hands.	Reduces transmission of microorganisms.
16. Record and report procedure in nurse's notes, mentioning specifically condition of oral cavity.	Documents response of client to hygiene measures.

Nurse Alert

Brushing is often contraindicated in clients who have undergone oral surgery or sustained trauma to the mouth. Avoid long-term use of lemon-glycerine swabs, since they can cause drying and shrinking of mucous membranes and gums, exhaustion of the salivary reflex, and erosion of tooth enamel.

Client Teaching

The client may be weak and unable to assist in his own care. However, the nurse can still provide instructions and answer any questions. She should discuss guidelines in the prevention of tooth decay: reducing intake of carbohydrates between meals, brushing within 30 minutes of eating sweets, always rinsing the mouth thoroughly with water, brushing and flossing before bedtime, and using fluoridated water if available.

Pediatric Considerations

A child's toothbrush should be approximately 21 cm (6 inches) in length.

Geriatric Considerations

Elderly persons can have reduced gum vascularity, decreased periodontal tissue elasticity, and brittle thin teeth. They also may have jaw bone atrophy. However, maintenance of regular dental hygiene should minimize periodontal disease.

Mouth Care for an Unconscious Client

The unconscious client poses special problems for the nurse with respect to mouth care. Many such clients have an absent or diminished gag reflex. Thus secretions tend to accumulate in the mouth, increasing the risk of aspiration. Critically ill clients often require an artificial airway and/or nasogastric tubes. These devices can cause considerable irritation to sensitive oral mucosal structures. Unconscious clients will require frequent mouth care to keep the mucosa well hydrated and intact.

Potential Nursing Diagnoses

The unconscious client in need of mouth care may have any one of the following nursing diagnoses:

    Actual or potential impairment of oral mucosal integrity related to retained secretions and/or local irritation

    Potential for injury related to absent gag reflex

    Alteration in comfort related to oral mucosal irritation

Equipment

Mouthwash or antiseptic solution
Toothettes or tongue blade wrapped in single layer of gauze
Padded tongue blade
Face towel
Emesis basin
Paper towels
Water glass with cool water
Petrolatum jelly
Suction catheter attached to suction

Steps	Rationale
1. Explain procedure to client.	Although unconscious, he may retain ability to hear explanation.
2. Wash your hands.	Reduces transmission of microorganisms.
3. Place paper towels on overbed table and arrange equipment.	Provides easy access to equipment.
4. Pull curtain around bed or close door to room.	Provides privacy.
5. Raise bed to its highest horizontal level. Lower side rail.	Use of good body mechanics prevents injury to both you and client.
6. Position client on side near you. Make sure that his head is turned toward mattress.	Protects client from aspirating secretions.
7. Place towel under client's face and emesis basin under his chin.	Prevents soiling of bed linen.
8. Carefully separate client's upper and lower teeth with padded tongue blade.	Prevents client from biting down on your fingers and provides access to oral cavity.
9. Clean client's mouth using toothettes or tongue blade moistened with mouthwash or water. Suction as needed during cleansing. Clean chewing and inner surfaces first. Swab roof of mouth and inside cheeks and lips. Swab tongue but avoid causing gag reflex if present. Moisten a clean applicator with water and swab mouth to rinse. Repeat as needed.	Swabbing stimulates gums and helps remove large food particles when brushing is impossible. Water or mouthwash provides lubricant for dry mucosa. Rinsing helps remove secretions and food particles. Suctioning minimizes risk of aspiration in clients with reduced gag reflex.

Steps	Rationale
10. Apply petrolatum jelly to client's lips.	Prevents lips from drying and cracking.
11. Explain to client that you have completed procedure.	Hearing and responsive capability are often still intact even in unconscious clients.
12. Reposition client comfortably, raise side rail, and return bed to its original position.	Maintains client's comfort and safety.
13. Clean equipment and return it to proper place. Dispose of soiled linen in "dirty" utility room.	Prevents spread of infection.
14. Wash your hands.	Reduces transmission of microorganisms.
15. Record and report procedure in nurse's notes, mentioning pertinent observations (e.g., presence of bleeding gums, dry mucosa, or crusts on tongue).	Accurate documentation should be timely and descriptive.

Nurse Alert

To ensure that any secretions in the client's pharynx are not aspirated, it may be helpful to have a second nurse assist with suctioning. Avoid the use of lemon glycerine swabs, which can cause drying of the mucosa and loss of tooth enamel.

Geriatric Considerations

With aging there is reduced vascularity of the gums. In elderly persons the teeth may be brittle, drier, and darker in color. If dental hygiene is not maintained, inflammation and swelling of periodontal tissues can easily occur.

Flossing Teeth

Brushing alone will not remove plaque and tartar from the surfaces of teeth. Inflammation of the gums (gingivitis), commonly caused by the formation of plaque and tartar along the gum line, is the most common dental problem among adults. Serious gum disease can lead to loss of teeth and painful mouth conditions.

Flossing mechanically removes plaque and tartar from tooth enamel. The nurse should encourage clients to floss daily for good preventive dental care.

Potential Nursing Diagnoses

The nurse will either assist clients in flossing or instruct them in the proper flossing technique. Potential diagnoses may include

Self-care deficit: hygiene, related to physical restrictions
Knowledge deficit regarding dental hygiene

Equipment

Dental floss (waxed or unwaxed)
Glass with water
Emesis basin
Mirror (optional)

Steps	Rationale
1. Wash hands.	Reduces transfer of microorganisms.
2. Pull curtain around bed or close room door.	Provides for client's privacy.
3. Position client supine with head of bed elevated, or he can be sitting.	Provides easy access to oral cavity.
4. Position overbed table in front of client and adjust mirror.	Client can comfortably view procedure.
5. Use 12-18 inches of floss wrapped around your index or middle fingers of both hands to hold taut a section ½-1 inch long. (Fig. 128)	Taut floss is easier to place between teeth.
6. To clean lower teeth, hold floss so forefingers of both your hands are on top of strand. Gently push floss between two teeth and work it in wide sweeping side-to-side arc. (Fig. 129)	Ensures removal of plaque and tartar as well as food particles from between teeth.
7. Carefully move floss up and down between tooth surfaces. Be sure that it slides both under gum	Removes plaque and tartar from tooth enamel. Thicker layers of plaque and tartar form at and below gumline.

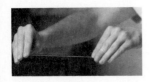

Fig. 128

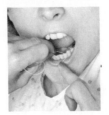

Fig. 129

Steps	Rationale
line and up toward biting surfaces. Repeat this motion two or three times. Also be sure to clean outer surfaces of the back molars.	
8. To clean upper teeth, hold floss over thumb of one hand and forefinger of other. Insert and move floss as on lower teeth. Repeat until teeth on both sides are clean.	Thumb helps to retract and support cheek.
9. As floss becomes frayed, move to another part of floss by unwinding part that is around your fingers.	Frayed floss becomes caught and can be torn off and lodged between teeth, causing gum inflammation and infection.
10. Allow client to rinse his mouth.	Removes debris from oral cavity.
11. Clean equipment and return to proper place. Wash hands.	Proper disposal reduces spread of infection.
12. Record procedure in nurse's notes, reporting any continued bleeding at gum line.	Documents client's response to hygienic care.

Nurse Alert

Clients with bleeding disorders are at risk of bleeding near the gum line. Confer with the physician to determine if flossing should be deferred.

Client Teaching

Allow the client an opportunity to practice flossing independently. Stress the importance of regular brushing in conjunction with flossing as part of a dental hygiene program.

Pediatric Considerations

The school-age child should begin to learn how to perform flossing daily. During school age the permanent teeth erupt.

Geriatric Considerations

Some elderly persons may have difficulty grasping and manipulating the floss. There are commercial floss holders available.

Shampooing Hair
in Bed

A client confined to bed should have regular shampooing to maintain the integrity of hair and scalp and to promote self-esteem and a sense of comfort. Staying in bed for several days results in the accumulation of excess oil and perspiration on the hair and scalp. Treatments may leave blood or solutions on the hair. The frequency of shampooing should depend on the condition of the hair and the client's daily routines.

Shampooing can be therapeutic in removing dried blood or gravel or dirt that could cause infection. Such debris is common in clients who have suffered head trauma or been in an accident. Medicated shampoos may be used when clients have specific hair or scalp problems. The nurse has an excellent opportunity to thoroughly assess the client's hair and scalp during shampooing.

Potential Nursing Diagnoses

Clients who require shampooing in bed may have any of the following nursing diagnoses:

Impairment in scalp related to trauma and/or dandruff
Self-care deficit: grooming, related to physical restrictions
Disturbance in self-concept related to appearance of hair

Equipment

Two bath towels
Face towel or washcloth
Shampoo (hair conditioner and cream rinse optional)

Water pitcher
Plastic trough
Washbasin
Bath blanket
Waterproof pad
Clean comb and brush
Hair dryer
Container of equal parts saline and hydrogen peroxide (optional)

Steps	Rationale
1. Explain to client what you are going to do.	Client may be apprehensive about positioning or risk of water entering his eyes.
2. Wash hands.	Reduces transfer of microorganisms.
3. Arrange equipment in a convenient place.	
4. Place a waterproof pad under client's shoulders, neck, and head. Position client with head and shoulders at top edge of bed. Place a plastic trough under client's head and a washbasin at end of	Prevents soiling of bed linen. Trough allows water to drain away from client's face into washbasin.

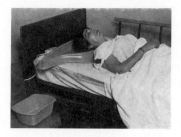

Fig. 130

Steps	Rationale
trough, being sure that trough extends beyond edge of mattress. (Fig. 130)	
5. Place rolled towel under client's neck and bath towel across his shoulders.	Prevents water from draining down back of client's neck.
6. Brush and comb client's hair.	Removing tangles results in more thorough cleaning.
7. Obtain water at 110° F (43°-44° C).	Prevents burns to scalp.
8. Ask client to hold a face towel or washcloth over his eyes.	Prevents soapsuds or water from entering eyes.
9. With water pitcher, slowly pour water over client's hair until it is completely wet. Apply a small amount of shampoo.	Water aids in distribution of shampoo suds over hair.
10. Work up a lather with both hands. Start at client's hairline and work toward back of neck. Lift head slightly with one hand to wash back of head. Massage scalp by applying pressure with your fingertips. Use peroxide and saline mixture to loosen any blood.	Massage increases scalp circulation.
11. Rinse hair with water. Make sure that water drains into basin. Repeat rinsing until client's hair is free of soap.	Retained soap leaves a dull finish on hair. Soap may cause scalp irritation.
12. Repeat Steps 9 through 11.	

Steps	Rationale
13. Apply conditioner if requested and rinse hair thoroughly.	Conditioner prevents excess drying. Cream rinse makes combing and brushing easier after drying.
14. Wrap client's head in bath towel. Dry his face with cloth that was used to protect his eyes.	Prevents dripping of water on client's skin and bed linen.
15. Dry client's hair and scalp. Use second towel if the first becomes saturated.	In clients who are ill, retained moisture may cause cooling and chills.
16. Comb his hair to remove tangles and dry it as quickly as possible.	Drying hair prevents chilling.
17. Assist client to a comfortable position.	
18. Return equipment to its proper place. Discard any disposable equipment and place soiled linen in "dirty" utility room. Wash your hands.	Maintains cleanliness of the client's immediate environment and controls transmission of infection.
19. Record in nurse's notes procedure accomplished and report any observations (e.g., lesions, dry flaky scalp, localized areas of inflammation).	Accurate documentation should be timely and descriptive of client's response and should include pertinent observations.

Nurse Alert

Shampooing may be contraindicated when the client has open incisions of the face, head, or neck. It may also be prohibited in the presence of cervical injuries, a tracheostomy, severe facial edema, or respiratory distress.

Client Teaching

Clients with scalp problems such as dandruff or pediculosis (lice) may require special instruction on the use of medicated shampoos or soaps.

Pediatric Considerations

An infant's or small child's hair may be shampooed while he is immersed in a basin or small tub during the bath. An infant's scalp usually is not excessively soiled and thus can be cleaned with mild soap and water. Never apply pressure directly over the infant's fontanels. For infants with cradle cap, loosen the scaly patches first with a small amount of oil and then wash gently.

Geriatric Considerations

A reduction in sebaceous gland secretion causes the hair of elderly persons to be less oily. Shampooing may be needed less frequently.

Making an Occupied Bed

Ill clients spend considerable time in bed—eating, bathing, using bedpans or urinals, and undergoing numerous therapeutic procedures. A bed should thus be kept as clean and comfortable as possible. At times it is necessary to make a bed when it is occupied by the client. He may be too weak to get out of bed, restricted from sitting in a chair by the nature of his illness, or confined by the presence of an external device such as a cast.

Making an occupied bed is difficult because it is harder to keep newly applied linen smooth and wrinkle free. The procedure can be done quickly, however, if the nurse organizes her actions effectively and has the client participate as much as possible with proper turning.

Potential Nursing Diagnoses

The nature of the procedure does not clearly dictate the use of specific nursing diagnoses. However, a client may likely be diagnosed as having

Impaired physical mobility related to imposed bedrest

Equipment

Linen bag	Top sheet (flat)
Bath blanket	Blanket
Mattress pad (needed only if other soiled)	Bedspread
	Waterproof pad(s)
Bottom sheet (fitted or flat)	Pillow case(s)
Draw sheet	Bedside chair or table

Steps	Rationale
1. Review client's chart for orders or specific precautions for movement and positioning.	Ensures safety of both you and client as well as proper use of body mechanics during procedure.
2. Explain procedure to client and assess client's physical capability to move.	Explanation promotes client cooperation during bedmaking.
3. Wash hands.	Reduces transmission of infection.
4. Assemble equipment and arrange it for convenience on bedside chair. Remove all unnecessary equipment (e.g., bedside table).	Planning and assembling equipment provide for smooth flow of procedure and ensure client's comfort. Placing linen on a clean surface minimizes spread of infection.
5. Provide privacy by drawing curtain or closing door.	Ensuring client's mental comfort is as important as ensuring his physical comfort.
6. Lower side rail on your side of bed. Remove call light.	Provides easy access to bed and linen.
7. Adjust bed height to comfortable working position. Assist client to supine or as flat a position as possible (unless he is short of breath).	Client's position promotes his comfort throughout procedure.
8. Loosen top sheet at foot of bed.	Makes it easier to remove.
9. Remove bedspread and blanket separately. Place them in linen bag if they are not to be reused. If they are to be reused, fold them in following manner: Bring top and bottom edges together.	This folding method facilitates replacement and prevents wrinkling.

Steps	Rationale
Fold side farther from your working side over onto nearer side. Bring top and bottom edges together again. Place folded linen over back of chair.	
10. Cover client with bath blanket in following manner: Unfold bath blanket over top sheet. Ask client to hold bath blanket. If client is unable to assist, tuck top of bath blanket under his shoulder. Grasp top sheet under bath blanket at client's shoulders and bring sheet down to foot of bed. Remove sheet and discard it in linen bag. (Fig. 131)	Bath blanket provides warmth and privacy during linen removal.
11. With assistance from another nurse, slide mattress toward head of bed.	If mattress slides toward foot of bed when head of bed is raised, it is difficult to tuck linen and is uncomfortable for client.

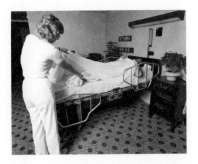

Fig. 131

Steps	Rationale
12. Position client on his side on far side of bed, facing away from you. Adjust pillow under his head.	Moving client provides space for placement of clean linen.
13. Loosen bottom linens, moving from head to foot of bed. Fan fold bottom linens toward client, first drawsheet and then bottom sheet. Tuck edges of linen just under client's buttocks, back, and shoulders. Do not fan fold mattress pad if it is to be reused. (Fig. 132)	This method provides maximum work space for placing clean linen.
14. If there is moisture on mattress, wipe off with towel and disinfectant.	Reduces transmission of infection.
15. Apply clean linen to exposed half of bed. ■ Place clean mattress pad on bed by unfolding it lengthwise with center crease in middle of bed. Fan fold top layer toward client and smooth the bottom	Applying linen over bed in successive layers minimizes energy needed during bedmaking.

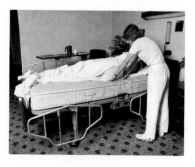

Fig. 132

Steps	Rationale
layer over mattress. (If pad is to be reused, simply smooth out wrinkles.)	
▪ Unfold bottom sheet lengthwise so center crease is lengthwise along center of bed. Fan fold sheet's top layer toward center of bed alongside client. Smooth the bottom layer of sheet over mattress and bring edge toward side at which you are standing. Allow it to hang about 25 cm (10 inches) over mattress edge. Lower hem of bottom sheet should lie seam down, even with bottom edge of mattress. (Fig. 133)	Proper positioning of linen on one side ensures that adequate linen will be available to cover opposite side of bed. Keeping seam edges down eliminates a source of irritation to client's skin.
16. Miter bottom sheet at head of bed.	Mitered corner is not loosened easily.
▪ Face head of bed diagonally. Place your hand under top corner of	

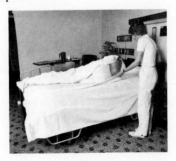

Fig. 133

Steps	Rationale

mattress near mattress edge and lift.

- Tuck top edge of bottom sheet smoothly under mattress so edges of sheet above and below mattress would meet if brought together.

- Face side of bed and pick up top edge of sheet approximately 45 cm (18 inches) from top of mattress.

- Lift sheet and lay it on top of mattress to form a triangular fold, with lower base of triangle even with mattress edge.

- Tuck lower edge of sheet, which is hanging free below mattress, under mattress. Tuck with palms down.

  Tucking sheets palms down prevents fingernails from catching on bedsprings.

- Hold sheet covering side edge of mattress in place with one hand. With your other hand, pick up top of triangular linen fold and bring it down over side of mattress. Tuck this portion of sheet under mattress.

- Tuck remaining portion of sheet under mattress, keeping linen smooth.

  Folds of linen are a source of irritation against client's skin.

Steps	Rationale
17. Move from head to foot of bed. Open drawsheet so it unfolds in half. Lay center fold along middle of bed lengthwise.	Ensures that enough linen is available to cover opposite side of bed.
18. Position drawsheet so it will lie under client's buttocks and torso. Fan fold top layer toward client with edge alongside client's back. Smooth the bottom layer out over mattress and tuck excess edge under mattress (keep palms down).	Drawsheet is used to lift and reposition client. Placement under torso distributes most of client's body weight over sheet.
19. Place waterproof pad over drawsheet with center fold against client's side. Fanfold top half toward client.	Used to protect bed linen from soiling.
20. Raise side rail on working side and go to other side of bed. Lower side rail there.	Maintains client safety during turning.
21. Assist client to roll slowly onto his other side, over folds of linen.	Exposes opposite side of bed for removal of soiled linen and placement of clean linen.
22. Loosen edges of soiled linen from underneath mattress.	
23. Remove soiled linen by folding it into a bundle with soiled side turned in. Discard it in linen bag.	Reduces transmission of microorganisms.
24. Spread clean fan-folded linen smoothly over edge of mattress from head to foot of bed.	Smooth linen prevents skin irritation.

Steps	Rationale
25. Assist client in rolling back into supine position. Reposition pillow.	Client comfort is maintained.
26. Miter top corner of bottom sheet (see Step 16). When tucking corner, be sure that sheet is taut.	Taut sheet eliminates wrinkles and folds that can irritate client's skin.
27. Facing side of bed, grasp remaining edge of bottom sheet. Lean back and pull to tuck excess linen tightly under mattress. Proceed from head to foot of bed. (Avoid lifting mattress to ensure a tight fit.)	Prevents wrinkles in bed linen.
28. Smooth the drawsheet over bottom sheet. Grasp edge of sheet with palms down, lean back, and tuck sheet tightly under mattress. Tuck from middle to top and then to bottom.	
29. Place top sheet over client with center fold lengthwise down middle of bed. Open sheet from head to foot and unfold it over client.	Ensures equal distribution of sheet over bed.
30. Ask client to hold clean top sheet, or tuck sheet around client's shoulders. Remove bath blanket and discard it into linen bag.	Sheet prevents exposure of body parts. Having client hold sheet encourages his participation.
31. Place blanket on bed, unfolding it so crease runs lengthwise along middle	Blanket should be placed to cover client completely and provide adequate warmth.

Steps	Rationale
of bed. Unfold blanket so it covers client. Top edge should be parallel with edge of top sheet and 15-20 cm (6-8 inches) down from top sheets edge.	
32. Apply bedspread in same manner as blanket (Step 31). Be sure that top edge of spread extends 2.5 cm (1 inch) above blanket's edge. Tuck top edge of spread over top edge of blanket.	Bedspread provides added warmth for client (who may require only a blanket).
33. Make a cuff by turning top edge of sheet down over edge of blanket and spread.	Smooth cuff protects client's face from irritation of rubbing on blanket.
34. At foot of bed, lift mattress corner slightly with one arm and tuck top linens under mattress. Top sheet, blanket, and bedspread are tucked under together. Be sure that linens are loose enough to allow movement of client's feet.	Pressure sores can develop on toes and heels if client's feet rub between tight-fitting bedsheets.
35. Make a modified mitered corner from top sheet and blanket: Pick up edge of blanket and top sheet approximately 45 cm (18 inches) from foot of mattress. Lift blanket and top sheet to form a triangular fold and lay it on bed. With one hand, hold linen already tucked under mat-	Modified mitered corner secures top linen but keeps even edge of blanket and top sheet draped over mattress.

Steps	Rationale
tress. With other hand, tuck loose edge hanging down under side of mattress. Pick up triangular fold and bring it down over mattress, holding linen in place on side of mattress. Do not tuck.	
36. Raise side rail. Make other side of bed, repeating Steps 34 and 35.	Side rail prevents client from accidentally falling out of bed.
37. Change pillowcase: Remove soiled case and discard it into linen bag with one hand. Grasp a clean pillowcase at center of closed end. Gather case, turning it inside out over hand holding it. With same hand, pick up middle of one end of pillow. Pull pillowcase down over pillow with other hand.	This method makes it easy to slide the case smoothly over the pillow.
38. Supporting client's head, place pillow under it.	Prevents hyperextension of neck.
39. Place call light within client's reach and return bed to a comfortable position.	Provides comfort and safety.
40. Open room curtains. Rearrange furniture. Place personal items within easy reach on overbed table or bedside stand.	Neat environment promotes a sense of well-being.
41. Discard dirty linen in linen hamper.	Prevents transmission of microorganisms.
42. Wash your hands.	

Client Teaching

During bedmaking there is considerable time that the nurse may use to discuss any topic with a client.

Geriatric Considerations

Elderly clients at risk of incontinence should have waterproof pads on the bed so excessive linen changes do not become necessary.

ELIMINA-
TION

Female Urinary Catheterization: Indwelling and Straight

Catheterization of the bladder involves the introduction of a rubber or plastic tube through the urethra into the bladder. The catheter provides for a continuous flow of urine in clients unable to control micturition or in those with obstruction to urinary outflow. Because in female clients the urethra is close to the anus, the risk of infection is always great and thorough cleaning of the perineum before catheter insertion is vital. Thereafter, frequent perineal care must be provided.

Potential Nursing Diagnoses

Clients who require insertion of a urinary catheter may have one or more of the following nursing diagnoses:

Altered urinary elimination related to incontinence

Altered urinary elimination related to urinary obstruction

Altered urinary elimination related to loss of voluntary bladder control

Equipment

Sterile catheterization tray

Sterile gloves

Sterile drapes, one fenestrated

Lubricant

Antiseptic cleansing solution

Cotton balls or gauze sponges

Forceps

Straight or indwelling catheter

    Prefilled syringe with solution to inflate balloon for in-
        dwelling catheter
    Receptacle or basin (usually bottom of tray)
    Specimen container
Flashlight or gooseneck lamp
Sterile drainage tubing and collection bag
Tape, rubber band, and safety pin
Bath blanket
Waterproof pad
Trash bag
Basin with warm water and soap
Bath towel

Steps	Rationale
1. Explain procedure to the client.	Minimizes client's anxiety and promotes cooperation.
2. Stand on left side of bed if you are right handed (or on right side if left handed). Clear bedside table and arrange equipment.	Successful catheter insertion requires that you assume a comfortable position with all equipment easily accessible.
3. Close cubicle or room curtains.	Reduces client's embarassment and aids in relaxation during procedure.
4. Place waterproof pad under client.	Prevents soiling of bed linen.
5. Assist client to a dorsal recumbent position (supine with knees flexed). Ask client to relax thighs so as to externally rotate them.	Provides good access to perineal structures.
6. Drape client with bath blanket. Place blanket diamond fashion over client: one corner at neck, one corner over each foot, and last corner over perineum.	Unnecessary exposure of body parts is avoided and client's comfort is maintained.

Steps	Rationale
7. Wash perineal area with soap and water as needed, and dry.	Presence of microorganisms near urethral meatus is reduced.
8. Wash your hands.	Transmission of bacteria from your hands is prevented.
9. If inserting indwelling catheter, open drainage system. Place drainage bag over edge of bottom bed frame. Bring drainage tube up between side rail and mattress.	Once catheter is inserted, you must immediately connect drainage system. Easy access prevents possible contamination. System is positioned to promote gravity drainage.
10. Position lamp to illuminate perineal area. (When using a flashlight, have another nurse hold it.)	Permits accurate identification and good visualization of urethral meatus.
11. Open catheterization kit according to directions, keeping bottom of container sterile.	Transmission of microorganisms from table or work area to sterile supplies is prevented.
12. Don sterile gloves (Skill 5-6).	Allows you to handle sterile supplies.
13. Pick up solid sterile drape by one corner and allow it to unfold. Be sure that it does not touch a contaminated surface.	Sterility of drape to be used as work surface is maintained.
14. Allow top edge of drape to form a cuff over both your hands. Place drape down on bed between client's thighs. Slip cuffed edge just under client's buttocks, taking care not to touch a contaminated surface with your gloves.	Outer surface of drape covering hands remains sterile. Sterile drape against sterile gloves is sterile.

Steps	Rationale
15. Pick up fenestrated sterile drape and allow it to unfold as in Step 13. Apply drape over client's perineum, exposing labia and being careful not to touch a contaminated surface.	Fenestrated drape provides a clean work area near catheter insertion site.
16. Place sterile trap and its contents on sterile drape between client's thighs.	Easy access to supplies during catheter insertion is provided.
17. Open packet containing antiseptic cleaning solution and pour contents over sterile cotton balls or gauze. (Be sure not to pour solution in receptacle that is to receive urine.)	All equipment is prepared before handling catheter to maintain aseptic technique during procedure.
18. Open urine specimen container, keeping top sterile.	Prepared to receive specimen.
19. Apply lubricant to bottom 2.5-5 cm (1-2 inches) of catheter tip.	Lubricant allows easy insertion of catheter tip through urethral meatus.

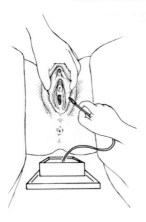

Fig. 134

Steps	Rationale
20. With your nondominant hand, carefully retract labia to fully expose urethral meatus. Maintain this position of your nondominant hand throughout remainder of procedure. (Fig. 134)	Full visualization of meatus is provided. Full retraction prevents contamination of meatus during cleansing. Closure of labia during cleansing requries that procedure be repeated.
21. With your dominant hand, pick up a cotton ball with forceps and clean perineal area, wiping front to back from clitoris toward anus. Use a new clean cotton ball for each wipe: along near labial fold, directly over meatus, and along far labial fold.	Cleaning reduces number of microorganisms at urethral meatus. Using single cotton ball for each wipe prevents transfer of microorganisms. Preparation moves from area of least contamination to area of most contamination. Your dominant hand remains sterile.
22. With your dominant hand, pick up catheter approximately 7.5 to 10 cm (3 to 4 inches) from the tip. Place the end of catheter in the urine tray receptacle.	Collection of urine prevents soiling of client's bed linen and allows accurate measurement of urinary output. Holding catheter near tip allows easier manipulation during insertion into meatus.

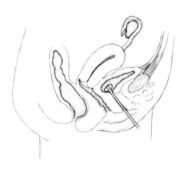

Fig. 135

Steps	Rationale
23. Ask client to bear down gently as if to void and slowly insert catheter through meatus.	Relaxation of external sphincter aids in insertion of the catheter.
24. Advance catheter approximately 5-7.5 cm (2-3 inches) in adult, 2.5 cm (1 inch) in child, or until urine flows out catheter end. When urine appears, advance catheter another 1.2 cm (½ inch).	Female urethra is short. Appearance of urine indicates that catheter tip is in bladder or lower urethra. Further advancement of catheter ensures bladder placement.
25. Release labia and hold catheter securely with your nondominant hand.	Bladder or sphincter contraction may cause accidental expulsion of catheter.
26. Collect urine specimen as needed: ▪ Fill specimen cup or jar to desired level (20-30 ml) by holding end of catheter in your nondominant hand over cup. With your dominant hand, pinch catheter to stop urine flow temporarily. Release catheter to allow remaining urine in bladder to drain into collection tray. Cover specimen cup and set it aside for labeling.	
27. Allow bladder to empty fully (unless institutional policy restricts maximal volume of urine to drain with each catheterization).	Retained urine may serve as reservoir for growth of microorganisms. (Caution must be taken to avoid hypotension resulting from sudden release of pressure against pelvic floor blood vessels.)

Steps	Rationale
28. With straight single-use catheter, withdraw it slowly but smoothly until removed.	Discomfort to client is minimized.
29. With indwelling catheter:	
■ While holding with thumb and little finger of your nondominant hand at meatus, take end of catheter and place it between first two fingers of that hand.	Catheter should be anchored while syringe is manipulated.
■ With your free dominant hand, attach syringe to injection port at end of catheter.	Port connects to lumen leading to inflatable balloon.
■ Slowly inject total amount of solution. If client complains of sudden pain, aspirate back and advance catheter farther.	Balloon within bladder is inflated. If malpositioned in urethra, it will cause pain during inflation.
■ After inflating balloon fully, release catheter with your nondominant hand and pull gently to feel resistance.	Inflation of balloon anchors catheter tip in place above bladder outlet. (Fig. 135)
30. Attach end of catheter to collecting tube of the drainage system.	Closed system for urine drainage is established.
31. Tape catheter to client's inner thigh with a strip of nonallergenic tape. Allow for slack so movement of thigh does not create tension on catheter.	Anchoring of catheter minimizes trauma to urethra and meatus during client movement. Nonallergenic tape prevents skin breakdown.

Steps	Rationale
32. Be sure that no obstructions or kinks are in tubing. Place excess coil of tubing on bed and fasten it to bottom bedsheet with a clip from drainage set or with rubber band and safety pin.	Patent tubing allows free drainage of urine by gravity and prevents backflow of urine into bladder.
33. Remove gloves and dispose of equipment, drapes, and urine in proper receptacles.	Transmission of microorganisms is prevented.
34. Assist client to a comfortable position. Wash and dry perineal area as needed.	Client comfort and security are maintained.
35. Instruct client on ways to position herself in bed with catheter: side lying facing drainage system—catheter and tubing on bed unobstructed; supine—catheter and tubing draped over thigh; side lying facing away from system—catheter and tubing extending between legs.	Urine should drain freely without obstruction. Placing catheter under extremities can result in obstruction due to compression of the tubing from client's weight. When the client is on one side facing away from system, catheter should not be placed over his upper thigh; this forces urine to drain uphill.
36. Caution client against pulling on catheter.	
37. Wash your hands.	Reduces transfer of microorganisms.
38. Record results of procedure in nurse's notes, including size of catheter, character of urine, and client's tolerance.	Documents client's response and results of therapy.

Nurse Alert

If the catheter is mistakenly introduced into the client's vagina, leave it in place. Open a new sterile catheter and place it in the urethra (which is immediately anterior to the vagina). Then remove the misplaced catheter.

Client Teaching

Instruct the client to keep the continuous drainage bag below the level of her bladder. This reduces the risk of urinary tract infections from backflow from the collection bag into the bladder. If the client is to be discharged with intermittent straight catheterization or with an indwelling (Foley) catheter, instruct her or a responsible person in catheter care, catheter insertion, and catheter removal.

Pediatric Considerations

Catheterization is most often used used when urethral obstruction or anuria due to renal failure is believed to be the cause of the child's failure to void. Most female infants and children accommodate an 8- or 10-gauge French catheter. Special care must be exercised to restrain and reassure the child during the procedure.

Geriatric Considerations

Foley catheters should not be used in an older client who is incontinent. The nurse must modify the client's fluid intake patterns and must adjust toileting procedures to acommodate to a routine that will maintain proper fluid balance, independence in toileting, and integrity of the perineal skin.

Male Urinary Catheterization: Indwelling and Straight

Catheterization of the bladder involves introduction of a rubber or plastic tube through the urethra and into the bladder. It is used for the following purposes: immediate relief of bladder distention, management of an incompetent bladder, obtaining a sterile urine specimen, and assessment of residual urine after voiding. Introduction of a catheter into a male client may be difficult if the prostate gland is enlarged. The nurse must not force a catheter through the urethra. She might cause tissue injury.

Potential Nursing Diagnoses

Clients requiring insertion of a catheter may have either or both of the following nursing diagnoses:

Altered urinary elimination related to urethral obstruction or incompetent bladder or to decreased level of consciousness

Self-care deficit: toileting, related to decreased mobility

Equipment

Sterile catheterization tray
Sterile gloves
Sterile drapes, one fenestrated
Lubricant
Antiseptic cleaning solution

Cotton ball or gauze sponges

Forceps

Straight or indwelling catheter

Prefilled syringe with solution to inflate balloon for indwelling catheter

Receptacle or basin (usually the bottom of tray)

Specimen container

Sterile drainage tubing and collection bag

Tape, rubber band, and safety pin

Bath blanket

Waterproof pad

Trash bag

Basin with warm water and soap

Bath towel

A flashlight or gooseneck lamp is not required in the catheterization of male clients.

Steps	Rationale
1. Explain procedure to client.	Minimizes client anxiety and promotes cooperation.
2. Stand on left side of bed if right handed, or on right side if left handed. Clear bedside table and arrange equipment.	Successful catheter insertion requires that you assume a comfortable position with all equipment easily accessible.
3. Close cubicle or room curtains.	Reduces client embarrassment and aids in relaxation during procedure.
4. Assist client to a supine position with thighs slightly abducted.	Prevents tensing of abdominal and pelvic muscles.
5. Drape client's upper trunk with bath blanket and cover lower extremities with bedsheets, exposing only genitalia.	Unnecessary exposure of body parts is prevented, and client comfort is maintained.
6. Place bath towel under genitalia.	Prevents soiling of bed linen.

Steps	Rationale
7. Wash perineum with soap and water as needed. In uncircumcised males, be sure to retract foreskin to clean urethral meatus. (Do *not* allow soap to get into meatus.)	Presence of microorganisms near urethral meatus is reduced.
8. Wash your hands.	Prevents transmission of bacteria from your hands to meatus.
9. If inserting an indwelling catheter, open drainage system. Place drainage bag over edge of bottom bed frame. Bring drainage tube up between side rail and mattress.	Once catheter is inserted, drainage system is immediately connected. Easy access prevents possible contamination. System is positioned to promote gravity drainage.
10. Open catheterization kit according to directions, keeping bottom of container sterile.	Transmission of microorganisms from table or work area to sterile supplies is prevented.
11. Don sterile gloves (Skill 5-6).	Maintains asepsis throughout procedure.
12. Apply sterile drapes. Pick up solid sterile drape by corner and allow it to unfold. Be sure that drape does not touch a contaminated surface. Apply drape over client's thighs just below penis. Pick up fenestrated sterile drape, allow it to unfold, and drape it over penis with fenestrated slit resting over glans.	Sterility of drape as work surface is maintained.
13. Place sterile tray and its contents on drape along-	Easy access to supplies during catheter insertion is provided.

Steps	Rationale
side client's thigh or on top of thighs.	
14. Obtain cotton balls or gauze with antiseptic solution. Open urine specimen container, keeping top sterile.	Prepares container for specimen.
15. Apply lubricant to bottom 12.5-17.5 cm (5-7 inches) of catheter tip.	Lubricant allows easy insertion of catheter tip through urethral meatus.
16. With your nondominant hand, retract foreskin of uncircumcised male. Grasp penis at shaft just below glans. Retract urethral meatus between thumb and forefinger. Maintain nondominant hand in this position throughout procedure.	Firm grasp minimizes chance that erection will occur (if an erection develops, discontinue procedure). Accidental release of foreskin or dropping of penis during cleaning requires process to be repeated.
17. With dominant hand, pick up a cotton ball with forceps and clean penis. Move it in a circular motion from meatus down to base of glans. Repeat cleaning two more times using a clean cotton ball each time.	Reduces number of microorganisms at meatus and moves from least contaminated to most contaminated area. Dominant hand remains sterile.
18. Pick up catheter with gloved dominant hand approximately 5-7.5 cm (2-3 inches) from catheter tip. Hold end of the catheter loosely coiled in the palm of your dominant hand (optional: grasp catheter with forceps).	Holding catheter near tip allows easier manipulation during insertion into meatus and prevents distal end from striking a contaminated surface.

Steps	Rationale
19. Lift penis to a position perpendicular to client's body and apply light traction. (Fig. 136)	Straightens urethral canal to ease catheter insertion.
20. Ask client to bear down as if to void and slowly insert catheter through meatus.	Relaxation of external sphincter aids in insertion of catheter.
21. Advance catheter 17.5-20 cm (7-8 inches) in an adult and 5-7.5 cm (2-3 inches) in a young child, or until urine flows out catheter end. If resistance is felt, withdraw catheter; do not force it through urethra. When urine appears, advance catheter another 1.2 cm (½ inch).	Adult male urethra is long. Appearance of urine indicates catheter tip is in bladder or urethra. Resistance to catheter passage may be caused by urethral strictures or enlarged prostate. Further advancement of catheter ensures proper placement.
22. Lower penis and hold catheter securely in non-	Catheter may be accidentally expelled by bladder or urethral

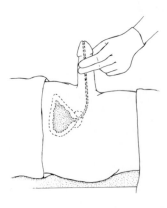

Fig. 136

Steps	Rationale
dominant hand. Place end of catheter in urine tray receptacle.	contraction. Collection of urine prevents soiling and provides output measurement.
23. Collect urine specimen according to Step 26 in female catheterization procedure (Skill 7-1).	
24. Allow bladder to empty fully (unless institutional policy restricts maximal volume of urine to drain with each catheterization).	Retained urine serves as reservoir for growth of microorganisms. (Precaution prevents hypotension resulting from sudden release of pressure against pelvic floor blood vessels under bladder.)
25. With straight single-use catheters, withdraw slowly but smoothly until removed. Replace foreskin over glans.	Minimizes discomfort during removal. Tightening of foreskin around shaft of penis can cause localized edema and discomfort.
26. With indwelling catheters, inflate balloon and check for proper anchoring as in Step 29 of Skill 7-1.	Ensures that tip will remain in place above bladder outlet. (Fig. 137)
27. Attach end of catheter to collecting tube of drainage system.	Establishes closed system for urine drainage.

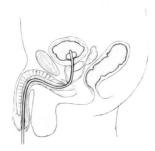

Fig. 137

Steps	Rationale
28. Tape catheter to client's inner thigh or lower abdomen (with penis directed toward client's chest). Use strip of nonallergenic tape. Provide slack so movement does not create tension on catheter.	Anchoring of catheter minimizes trauma to urethra and meatus. Taping to abdomen minimizes irritation at angle of penis and scrotum. Nonallergenic tape prevents skin breakdown.
29. Be sure that there are no obstructions or kinks in tubing. Place excess coil of tubing on bed and fasten it to bottom bedsheet with a clip to drainage set or with a rubber band and safety pin. (Fig. 138)	Patent tubing allows free drainage of urine by gravity and prevents backflow of urine into bladder.
30. Remove gloves and dispose of all equipment.	Prevents transmission of microorganisms.
31. Assist client to a comfortable position and wash and dry perineal areas as needed.	Promotes client comfort.

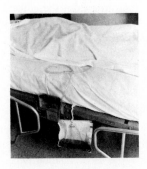

Fig. 138

Steps	Rationale
32. Instruct client on proper positioning and the importance of not pulling on catheter (see Steps 35 and 36 of Skill 7-1).	Ensures unobstructed drainage through a closed system.
33. Wash your hands.	Reduces transmission of microorganisms.
34. Record in nurse's notes results of procedure, including size of catheter, amount of urine drained, character of urine, and client's tolerance.	Documents client's response and results of therapy.

Nurse Alert

Do not force the catheter if resistance is met. In older men, prostatic hypertrophy may partially obstruct the urethra and prevent easy passage of the catheter. If resistance is met, notify the client's physician.

Client Teaching

Instruct the client to keep the continuous drainage bag below the level of his bladder. This reduces the risk of urinary tract infections due to backflow from the collection bag into the bladder. If the client is to be discharged with intermittent straight catheterization or with an indwelling Foley catheter, instruct him or his family on catheter care, insertion, and removal.

Pediatric Considerations

Male infants may not be able to accommodate the 8- or 10-gauge French catheters. In such instances a smaller soft plastic feeding tube may be used. Caution is necessary in catheterizing young males to avoid trauma that might result in sterility from damage to the ductal and glandular openings into the urethra.

Geriatric Considerations

Foley catheters should be avoided whenever possible in older adult clients who are incontinent. The nurse must modify the client's fluid intake patterns and schedule toileting procedures so a routine for bladder elimination will be developed that maintains proper fluid balance, independence in toileting, and skin integrity.

Applying a Condom Catheter

A condom catheter is an external urinary drainage device that is convenient to use and safe for draining urine in male clients. It is a soft pliable rubber sheath that slips over the penis, and it is suitable for incontinent or comatose clients who still have complete and spontaneous bladder emptying. The catheter may be preferred over an indwelling (Foley) type because drainage is maintained with less risk of infection.

Potential Nursing Diagnoses

Clients who require application of a condom catheter may have either or both of the following nursing diagnoses:

Altered urinary elimination related to incontinence

Self-care deficit: toileting, related to decreased level of consciousness

Equipment

Rubber condom sheath

Strip of elastic or Velcro adhesive

Urinary collection bag with drainage tubing

Basin with warm water and soap

Towel and washcloth

Bath blanket

Steps	Rationale
1. Wash hands.	Reduces transmission of microorganisms.
2. Explain procedure to client.	Reduces client anxiety and improves cooperation.
3. Assist client to a supine position. Place bath blanket over his upper trunk and cover his lower extremities with bedsheets so only the genitalia are exposed.	Supine position promotes comfort, and draping prevents unnecessary exposure of body parts.
4. Clean the genitalia with soap and water. Dry thoroughly.	Secretions that may irritate client's skin are removed. Rubber sheath rolls onto dry skin more easily.
5. Prepare urinary drainage bag by attaching it to bed frame. Bring drainage tubing up through side rails onto bed.	Easy access to equipment during connection of condom catheter is provided.
6. Grasp client's penis firmly along shaft with your nondominant hand. With your dominant hand, hold condom sheath at tip of penis and smoothly roll sheath up onto penile shaft.	Firm grasp reduces chances that erection will occur. Condom should fit smoothly to prevent sites of constriction.
7. Be sure that tip of penis is 2.5-5 cm (1-2 inches) above end of condom catheter.	Allows free passage of urine into collecting tubing during voiding.
8. Encircle penile shaft with strip of Velcro or elastic adhesive. Be sure that strip touches only condom sheath. Apply snugly but not tightly. (Fig. 139)	Adhesive strip anchors condom in place. Snug fit prevents constriction of blood flow.

Steps	Rationale
9. Connect drainage tubing to end of condom catheter.	Prevents soiling of bed linen and provides for collection of all voided urine.
10. Place excess coil of tubing on bed and secure to bottom bedsheet.	Patent tubing promotes free drainage of urine.
11. Dispose of soiled equipment and wash your hands.	Reduces transmission of microorganisms.
12. Record when condom catheter was applied and presence of urine in drainage bag.	Documents procedure. Also notes that client is able to empty his bladder and that urine is contained in drainage bag.

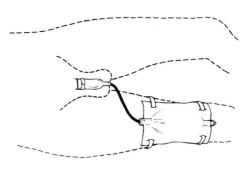

Fig. 139

Nurse Alert

Adhesive tape should never be used to secure a condom catheter. It can cause constriction and reduction of blood flow to the penis. Velcro or elastic adhesive expands with changes in size of the penis and does not reduce blood flow.

Client Teaching

Occasionally the client will return home and wear a condom catheter intermittently or throughout the day. Instruct him and his family in perineal care, catheter application, and use of the optional leg bag.

Pediatric Considerations

Pediatric urinary collection bags are applied to the male infant or child when exact urinary output is required. The adolescent male may be catheterized only if there is no other method of obtaining exact urinary output.

Geriatric Considerations

Older men may require more frequent bladder emptying and should be offered the urinal or taken to the bathroom more frequently rather than subjected to condom catheter application.

Administering an Enema

An enema is the instillation of a solution into the rectum and sigmoid colon. It is administered to promote defecation by stimulating peristalsis. Medications are occasionally given by enema to exert a local effect on the rectal mucosa. A cleansing enema can be used to soften feces that have become impacted or to empty the rectum and lower colon for diagnostic or surgical procedures.

Potential Nursing Diagnoses

Clients who require an enema may have one or more of the following nursing diagnoses:

Altered bowel elimination: constipation, related to immobility or improper diet

Altered bowel elimination related to medications

Self-care deficit: toileting, related to loss of voluntary muscle control

Equipment

Administration via rectal tube with container

Enema container

Ordered volume of solution warmed to 40.5°-43° C (105°-109° F) (with soap, salt, or other additives)

Rectal tube with rounded tip

Tubing to connect rectal tube to container

Regulating clamp on tubing

Bath thermometer to measure solution's temperature

Lubricating jelly

Waterproof pad

Bath blanket

Toilet paper

Bedpan or commode
Washcloth and towel
Disposable gloves
Administration via prepackaged disposable container
Prepackaged bottle with rectal tip
Disposable gloves
Lubricating jelly
Waterproof pad
Bath blanket
Toilet paper
Bedpan or commode
Washcloth and towel

Steps	Rationale
Rectal Tube With Container	
1. Explain procedure to client.	Reduces client anxiety and promotes cooperation during procedure.
2. Close room or cubicle curtains.	Provides client privacy.
3. Assist client into a left side-lying (Sims) position with right knee flexed. Children may also be placed in dorsal recumbent position. (Position clients with poor sphincter control on bedpan.)	Allows enema solution to flow downward by gravity along natural curve of sigmoid colon and rectum, thus improving retention of solution. (Clients with poor sphincter control will not be able to retain all enema solution.)
4. Place waterproof pad under client's hips and buttocks.	Prevents soiling of bed linen.
5. Drape client's trunk and lower extremities with bath blanket, leaving only anal area exposed.	Prevents unnecessary exposure of body parts and reduces client embarrassment.
6. Assemble enema container—connecting tubing, clamp, and rectal	Rectal tubing should be small enough to fit diameter of client's anus but large enough

Steps	Rationale
tube. Size of rectal tube should be 10-12 gauge French for infant or child and 22-26 gauge French for adult.	to prevent leakage around tube.
7. Close regulating clamp.	Prevents initial loss of solution as it is added to container.
8. Add warmed solution to container. Warm the water as it flows from faucet. Place saline container in basin of hot water before adding saline to enema container. Check temperature of solution with bath thermometer or by pouring small amount of solution over your inner wrist.	Hot water can burn intestinal mucosa. Cold water can cause abdominal cramping and is difficult to retain.
9. Raise container, release clamp, and allow solution to flow enough to fill tubing.	Removes air from tubing.
10. Reclamp tubing.	Prevents further loss of solution.
11. Place bedpan near bedside unit.	To be easily accessible if client is unable to retain enema.
12. Wash your hands.	Reduces transmission of infection.
13. Don disposable gloves.	Prevents transmission of organisms from feces.
14. Lubricate 3-4 inches of tip of rectal tube with lubricating jelly.	Allows smooth insertion of tube without risk of irritation or trauma to rectal mucosa.

Maximum volumes for saline or tap water enemas (ml)

Infant	150-250
Toddler	250-350
School-age child	300-500
Adolescent	500-750
Adult	750-1000

Steps	Rationale
15. Gently separate buttocks and locate anus. Instruct client to relax by breathing out slowly through his mouth.	Breathing out promotes relaxation of external anal sphincter.
16. Insert tip of rectal tube slowly by pointing it in direction of client's umbilicus. Length of insertion varies: 7.5-10 cm (3-4 inches) for adult; 5-7.5 cm (2-3 inches) for child; 2.5-4 cm (1-1½ inches) for infant. Withdraw tube immediately if it meets obstruction.	Careful insertion prevents trauma to rectal mucosa from accidental lodging of tube against wall. Insertion beyond proper limit can cause bowel perforation.
17. Continue to hold tubing until end of fluid instillation.	Bowel contraction can cause expulsion of rectal tube.
18. Open regulating clamp and allow solution to enter slowly, with container at client's hip level.	Rapid infusion can stimulate evacuation prematurely before sufficient volume is infused.
19. Raise height of container slowly to appropriate level above anus (30-45 cm or 12-18 inches). Infusion time varies with volume of solution administered (e.g., 1 liter in 10 minutes).	Allows for continuous slow infusion. Raising container too high causes rapid infusion and possible painful distention of colon.
20. Lower the container or clamp tubing if client complains of cramping or if fluid escapes from anus around tube.	Temporary cessation of infusion prevents cramping. Cramping may prevent client from retaining all fluid.
21. Clamp tubing after all solution is infused.	Prevents entrance of air into rectum.

Steps	Rationale
22. Place layers of toilet tissue around tube at anus and gently withdraw tube.	Provides for client's comfort and cleanliness.
23. Explain to client that feeling of distention is normal. Ask him to retain solution as long as possible while lying quietly in bed. (For an infant or young child, gently hold buttocks together for a few minutes.)	Solution distends bowel. Length of retention varies with type of enema and client's ability to contract anal sphincter. Longer retention promotes more effective stimulation of peristalsis and defecation. (Infants and young children have poor sphincter control.)
24. Discard enema container and tubing in proper receptacle or rinse out thoroughly with warm water and soap if container is to be reused.	Controls transmission and growth of microorganisms.
25. Remove gloves by pulling them inside out and discard in proper receptacle.	Prevents microorganism transmission.
26. Assist client to bathroom or help position him on bedpan.	Normal squatting position promotes defecation.
27. Observe character of feces and solution (caution client against flushing toilet before inspection).	When enemas are ordered "until clear," it is essential to observe the contents of solution passed.
28. Assist client as needed to wash anal area with warm water and soap.	Fecal contents can irritate skin. Hygiene promotes client's comfort.
29. Wash your hands and record results of enema in nurse's notes.	Prompt recording improves documentation of treatment results.

Prepackaged Disposable Container

1. Follow Steps 1 through 5 of previous procedure.

Steps	Rationale
2. Place bedpan near bedside unit.	To be easily accessible if client unable to retain enema.
3. Wash your hands.	Reduces transmission of infection.
4. Don disposable gloves.	Prevents transmission of organisms from feces.
5. Remove plastic cap from rectal tip. Although tip is already lubricated, more jelly can be applied as needed.	Lubrication provides for smooth insertion of rectal tube without causing rectal irritation or trauma.
6. Gently separate buttocks and locate anus. Instruct client to relax by breathing out slowly through his mouth.	Breathing out promotes relaxation of external anal sphincter.
7. Insert tip of bottle gently into rectum. Advance it 7.5-10 cm (3-4 inches) in adult. (Children and infants usually do not receive prepackaged hypertonic enemas.) (Fig. 140)	Gentle insertion prevents trauma to rectal mucosa.
8. Squeeze bottle until all solution has entered rectum and colon. (Most bottles contain approximately 250 ml.)	Hypertonic solutions require only small volumes to stimulate defecation.
9. Follow Steps 22 through 29 of previous procedure.	

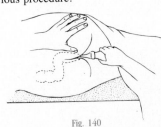

Fig. 140

Nurse Alert

If a client has an order for enemas "until clear," the nurse should not give more than three without verifying with the physician the need for more. Repeated enema administration can result in serious fluid and electrolyte imbalances.

Client Teaching

Clients should be instructed not to rely on enemas to maintain bowel regularity. Repeated use of enemas destroys defecation reflexes and leads to further alterations in bowel elimination.

Pediatric Considerations

The procedure for giving an enema to an infant or a child does not differ essentially from that for giving one to an adult. However, because of lack of motor control in the rectum, infants and small children may be unable to retain the instilled fluid. Plain tap water is rarely used in children because, being hypotonic, it can cause rapid fluid shifts and fluid overload. The Fleet enema is not advised for children because of the harsh action of its ingredients, which may produce severe diarrhea (leading to metabolic acidosis).

Geriatric Considerations

A frail elderly client may be more susceptible than a young adult client to fluid and electrolyte imbalances resulting from enema administration. Caution should be used when administering repeated cleansing enemas. In addition, the nurse should frequently monitor fluid and electrolyte status.

Removing Stool Digitally

Digital stool removal involves the introduction of the nurse's fingers into the client's rectum to break up a fecal mass and remove it in sections. This procedure is used when the fecal mass is too large to be passed voluntarily and enema administration is unsuccessful. Elderly or immobilized clients who are unable to ambulate regularly and who fail to maintain a balanced diet or fluid intake are susceptible to fecal impaction.

Potential Nursing Diagnoses

Clients who require digital stool removal may have either or both of the following nursing diagnoses:

Altered bowel elimination: constipation, related to fecal impaction

Impaired physical mobility

Equipment

Lubricant
Gloves
Bedpan
Waterproof pad
Bath blanket
Washcloth
Towel

Steps	Rationale
1. Measure client's pulse rate.	Serves as baseline for determining changes during procedure.
2. Explain procedure to client, noting that manipulation of the rectum can cause discomfort.	Explanation reduces client anxiety. Cooperation is necessary to minimize risk of injury.
3. Assist client to a side-lying position with knees flexed.	Provides access to rectum.
4. Drape client's trunk and lower extremities with bath blanket.	Prevents unnecessary exposure of body parts.
5. Place waterproof pad under client's buttocks.	Prevents soiling of bed linen.
6. Place bedpan next to client.	To be receptacle for stool.
7. Don disposable gloves.	Prevents transmission of microorganisms.
8. Lubricate your gloved index finger with ample amount of lubricating jelly.	Permits smooth insertion of finger into rectum.
9. Insert your finger into client's rectum and advance it slowly along rectal wall toward umbilicus.	Allows you to reach impacted stool high in rectum.
10. Gently loosen fecal mass by massaging around it. Work finger into hardened core.	Loosening mass allows you to penetrate it with less discomfort to client.
11. Work stool downward toward anus. Remove small sections of feces at a time.	Prevents need to force finger up into rectum and minimizes trauma to mucosa.

Steps	Rationale
12. Periodically assess client's heart rate and look for signs of fatigue. Stop procedure if client's heart rate drops or rhythm changes.	Vagal stimulation slows heart rate. Procedure may exhaust client.
13. Continue to clear rectum of feces and allow client to rest at intervals.	Rest improves client's tolerance of procedure.
14. After disimpaction, use washcloth and towel to wash buttocks and anal area.	Promotes client's sense of comfort and cleanliness.
15. Remove bedpan and dispose of feces. Remove gloves by turning them inside out and discard in proper receptacle.	Prevents transmission of microorganisms.
16. Assist client to toilet or a clean bedpan.	Disimpaction may stimulate defecation reflex.
17. Wash your hands and record in nurse's notes results of disimpaction. Describe fecal characteristics. (Procedure may be followed by enemas or cathartics.)	Prompt recording improves accuracy of documentation.

Nurse Alert

Excessive rectal manipulation can cause irritation to the mucosa, bleeding, and stimulation of the vagus nerve. When there is vagal stimulation, a reflexive slowing of the heart rate occurs and can cause dangerous arrhythmias in some clients.

Client Teaching

Clients and their families should be instructed how to avoid fecal impactions—by modifying their diets to include more fruits and vegetables, by increasing their fluid intake (if not contraindicated), and by altering sedentary activity patterns.

Pediatric Considerations

Digital removal of stool is rarely needed in children. If it does become necessary, it should be preceded by a careful explanation to both the parent and the child. Preventive measures are more common and include stool softeners, diet changes, and adequate hydration.

Geriatric Considerations

In the older adult population, constipation tends to be more a problem than in younger persons, and along with it the more frequent use of laxatives and/or enemas. In addition, there is a higher percentage of elderly clients with chronic cardiovascular disease, which puts these persons at greater risk of arrhythmias induced by vagal stimulation during digital stool removal.

CARE OF THE SURGICAL CLIENT

Demonstrating Postoperative Exercises

The manner in which the nurse prepares a client for surgery can have a positive influence on his recovery. With well-planned instruction a client can learn how to cough and deep breathe regularly, ambulate and resume activities of daily living early after surgery, and participate in the recovery process to attain a sense of well-being. A few simple maneuvers—diaphragmatic breathing, coughing, turning, and leg exercises—serve to prevent respiratory and circulatory complications that otherwise might develop in a client who stays inactive postoperatively. The exercises are important for any client undergoing general anesthesia.

Diaphragmatic breathing promotes lung expansion and helps clear respiratory passages of anesthetic gases. Coughing assists in removing retained mucus that accumulates in the airways because of depressed respirations and anesthesia. Leg exercises and turning improve blood flow to the lower extremities, thus reducing venous stasis.

When the nurse plans postoperative exercises, it is important to know the client's risks of complications. Chronic smoking, a history of respiratory disease, and a long surgical incision all can contribute to impairing a client's ventilatory capacity. Likewise, a history of peripheral vascular disease or forced immobilization from an applied cast or traction can increase the risk of poor circulatory perfusion. By helping clients learn how to participate actively in postoperative recovery the nurse provides an effective and preventive plan of care.

Potential Nursing Diagnoses

Clients undergoing surgery can have any of a number of nursing diagnoses. Potential diagnoses that have the greatest impact on a client's ability to perform postoperative exercises correctly may include:

Ineffective airway clearance related to incisional pain and/ or reduced consciousness

Alteration in comfort related to surgical incision

Impaired physical mobility related to pain and/or imposed restrictions of movement

Equipment

Pillow (optional)

Steps	Rationale
Diaphragmatic Breathing	
Demonstrate the following steps to client:	
1. Sit or stand upright, placing your hands palm down along lower borders of your anterior rib cage. (Fig. 141)	Upright position facilitates diaphragmatic excursion. This placement of hands allows individual to feel movement of chest and abdomen as diaphragm descends and lungs expand.

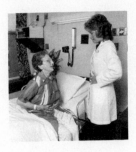

Fig. 141

Steps	Rationale
2. Take slow deep breath, inhaling through your nose.	Discourages panting or hyperventilation. Breathing through nose warms, humidifies, and filters air.
3. Give attention to normal downward movement of your diaphragm during inspiration. Abdominal organs descend, and thorax expands slowly.	Your explanation focuses on normal ventilatory movements so the client can anticipate how diaphragmatic breathing feels.
4. Avoid using your chest and shoulders while inhaling.	Use of auxiliary chest and shoulder muscles increases energy expenditure during breathing.
5. After holding your breath to a count of 3, slowly exhale through your mouth.	Allows gradual expulsion of all air.
6. Repeat exercise three to five times.	Establishes slow rhythmical breathing pattern.
7. Have client practice exercise.	Reinforces learning.

Coughing

Demonstrate the following steps to client:

1. Assume an upright position in bed or on side of bed.	Facilitates diaphragmatic movement and enhances expansion of lungs.
2. Take two or three slow diaphragmatic breaths.	Expands lungs fully to move air behind mucus in airways.
3. Inhale deeply, hold your breath to count of 3, and cough once and then again.	Two successive coughs help remove mucus more effectively and completely than one forceful cough.
4. Do not merely clear your throat.	Clearing of throat does not remove mucus from deep in airways.

Steps	Rationale
5. If surgical incision is to be in chest or abdominal area, place one hand over the incisional area and other hand on top of first. During inhalation and coughing, press gently against that area to splint incision. (A pillow over incision is optional.) (Fig. 142)	Surgical incision results in cutting of muscles and tissues. Breathing and coughing place strain on a suture line and cause discomfort. Splinting minimizes incisional pulling. Hands provide firm support to incision.
6. Have client practice coughing with splinting.	You are trying to emphasize value of deep coughing with splinting to effectively expectorate mucus with minimal discomfort.

Turning

NOTE: This is for turning client to his left side.

1. Instruct client to assume a supine position on right half of bed. (Side rails should be up on both sides.)	You cannot demonstrate exercise in client's bed for obvious reasons of asepsis. Positioning begins toward right side of bed so turning to left will not cause client to roll toward bed's edge.
2. Place client's left hand over incisional area for splinting.	Supports incisional area to minimize pulling of suture line during turning.

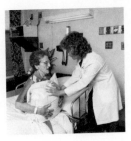

Fig. 142

Steps	Rationale
3. Have client keep his left leg straight and flex right knee up and over left leg.	Straight left leg stabilizes client's position. Flexed right leg shifts weight for easier turning.
4. Grasping side rail on left side of bed with his right hand, client pulls toward left and rolls onto his left side.	Minimizes effort needed to turn.

Leg Exercises

NOTE: If client's surgery involves one or both extremities, a surgeon's order is required before exercises can be performed postoperatively. Legs unaffected by surgery can be safely exercised unless a client has preexisting alterations.

Steps	Rationale
1. Place client supine in bed. Demonstrate leg exercises by putting him through passive range of motion.	Provides for normal anatomical position of lower extremities.
2. Instruct client to rotate each ankle in a complete circle by pretending to	Maintains joint mobility and promotes venous return.

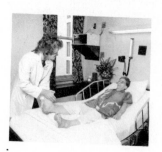

Fig. 143

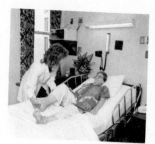

Fig. 144

Steps	Rationale

draw circles with his big toe. (Fig. 143)

3. Alternate dorsiflexion and plantar flexion of the feet. Client will feel his calf muscles first contract and then relax.

Stretches and contracts gastrocnemius muscles.

4. Have client flex and extend his knees. (Fig. 144)

5. Keeping his legs straight, client then alternately raises each leg from surface of bed and lets it drop gently.

Promotes contraction and relaxation of quadriceps muscles.

Nurse Alert

Know whether a client will be allowed to do active exercising of his extremities postoperatively. Some vascular procedures, such as repair of the femoral-popliteal artery, prohibit active exercising until the vascular graft has healed. Likewise, certain procedures may contraindicate turning.

Client Teaching

The nurse must demonstrate each exercise carefully and then have the client practice doing it under supervision. Eventually the client should be able to perform the exercises independently. During a routine postoperative day it is hoped that he will become able to initiate exercises on his own.

Pediatric Considerations

Children usually are at lower risk of postoperative complications because they tend to resume activity quickly. However, seriously ill children may require guidance and support. Parents can be helpful in demonstrating and reinforcing exercises.

Geriatric Considerations

Elderly persons usually are at greater risk of postoperative complications because of the aging process. They often have increased calcium and cholesterol deposits in small arteries, and vessel walls thicken. These changes predispose to clot formation. The elderly person's rib cage also tends to stiffen and diaphragmatic movement declines, reducing lung expansion. It often takes longer for an elderly client to become oriented following surgery due to neurological and sensory changes. Thus active participation in exercises may be lessened.

Shaving a Surgical Site: Wet Shave

Before any surgical procedure, the skin is prepared so the number of resident microorganisms that could enter a surgical wound will be minimized. Skin preparation routinely requires thorough cleaning with scrubs and/or showers. Shaving may also be performed to remove body hair that harbors microorganisms and obstructs the view of the surgical field. An area of skin larger than the actual surgical site is always prepared to ensure that the surgical site is as clean as possible.

Although some physicians order a preoperative shave the night before surgery, it is preferable to shave hair immediately before surgery. Hair removal can injure the skin, especially if a razor is used. Minor nicks or cuts in the skin are prime sites for bacterial growth. The longer the period between the shave and surgery, the greater is the potential for bacterial growth.

Potential Nursing Diagnoses

If the technique of shaving a surgical site is not performed correctly, injury to the skin may pose the following nursing diagnoses:

Potential for injury related to skin infection
Impaired skin integrity related to razor cuts
Alteration in comfort related to skin abrasions or cuts

Equipment

Portable lamp to illuminate site
Bath blanket for draping client

363

Wet shave
>   Razor with extra blade
>   Clean basin with warm water
>   Gauze sponges
>   Basin with liquid antiseptic soap mixed with water
>   Waterproof underpad or towels
>   Washcloth
>   Cotton balls, cotton-tipped applicator, and antiseptic so-
>   lution (optional)

Steps	Rationale
1. Wash hands.	Reduces transmission of microorganisms.
2. Refer to physician's order to determine portion of body to shave.	Shaving wide area around incision site further reduces risk of contamination by hair.
3. Provide for client's privacy by closing the room divider or door. Drape client. Leave only area to be shaved at one time (10-20 cm or 4-8 inches) exposed.	Promotes comfort and reduces anxiety.
4. Place towel or waterproof pad under body part to be shaved.	Prevents soiling of bed linen.
5. Lather client's skin with gauze sponges dipped in antiseptic soap.	Softens hair and reduces friction against skin from the razor.
6. Shave small area at time (approximately 10-20 cm). With your nondominant hand, gently stabilize skin. With razor held in your dominant hand at 45-degree angle, shave in same direction as hair grows. Use short gentle strokes. (Fig. 145)	Shaving small area minimizes cutting. Direction of shave prevents pulling of hair.

Steps	Rationale
7. Rinse razor as soap and hair accumulate on blade. Discard blades as they become dull.	Maintains clean razor edge to promote client's comfort.
8. Rearrange drapes as each portion of shave is completed.	Maintains client's comfort.
9. Use washcloth and warm water to remove hair and soap solution. Discard waterproof pad or towel.	Reduces skin irritation.
10. Observe skin for any nicks or cuts. Report them to physician.	Break in skin integrity increases the risk of infection.
11. Dispose of equipment according to agency policy.	Prevents spread of infection and reduces risk of injury from razor blades.
12. Record in nurse's notes area of skin prepared.	Documents procedure completed.
13. (Optional) When shaved area is over body crevices (e.g., umbilicus or groin), clean crevices with cotton-tipped applicators or cotton balls dipped in antiseptic solution. Dry with cotton balls or applicators.	Removes secretions, dirt, and any remaining hair clippings, which harbor microorganisms.

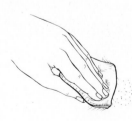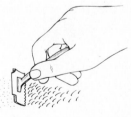

Fig. 145

Nurse Alert

Use extra caution if the client has a preexisting bleeding tendency such as leukemia, aplastic anemia, or hemophilia or has been receiving anticoagulant therapy. If a client has a bleeding tendency or is on anticoagulant therapy, dry shaving may be ordered.

Client Teaching

Explain the purpose of shaving and its importance to the client's welfare. The client should understand that it is necessary to shave a larger surface area than the immediate surgical site. He may fear that the surgical incision will be as large as the shaved area.

Pediatric Considerations

A shave will sometimes be deferred because the amount of body hair on a young child is limited. An adolescent has more body hair and may need to undergo a shave.

Geriatric Considerations

The elderly client's skin can be thin and fragile. Use caution when shaving to avoid cuts.

Shaving a Surgical Site: Dry Shave

As in the case of wet shaving, dry shaving removes hair that obstructs the view of the surgical field and harbors microorganisms. The Centers for Disease Control (CDC) recommends using clippers or a depilatory to remove hair so as to prevent cutting the client's skin. Small cuts or nicks are prime sites for bacterial growth.

If the client receives a skin scrub or shower prior to a dry shave, it is very important to dry the skin thoroughly before shaving. The clippers will not cut as effectively if the hair is wet.

Potential Nursing Diagnoses

The nurse will perform a dry shave for clients with a variety of nursing diagnoses. A dry shave does not pose identifiable diagnoses.

Equipment

Portable lamp to illuminate site
Bath blanket for draping client
Electric clippers
Scissors
Towel
Antiseptic solution, cotton balls, cotton-tipped applicators (optional)

Steps	Rationale
1. Wash hands.	Reduces transmission of microorganisms.
2. Refer to physician's order to determine portion of body to shave.	Shaving wide area around incision site further reduces risk of contamination by hair.
3. Provide for client's privacy by closing room curtains or door. Drape client. Leave only area to be shaved at one time (10-20 cm or 4-8 inches) exposed.	Promotes comfort and reduces anxiety.
4. Lightly dry area to be shaved with towel.	Eliminates moisture, which can interfere with clean cut of clippers.
5. Hold clippers approximately 1 cm above skin and shave in same direction as hair grows.	Prevents abrasion of skin and pulling of hair.
6. Rearrange drapes as necessary.	
7. Lightly brush off cut hair with towel.	Removes contaminated hair and promotes client's comfort.
8. Dispose of equipment according to agency policy.	Prevents spread of infection.
9. Record in nurse's notes area of skin prepared.	Documents that procedure was completed.
10. (Optional) When shaved area is over body crevices (e.g., umbilicus or groin), clean crevices with cotton-tipped applicators or cotton balls dipped in antiseptic solution. Dry with cotton balls or applicators.	Removes secretions, dirt, and any remaining hair clippings, which harbor microorganisms.

Client Teaching

Explain to the client the purpose of shaving. He should understand why it is necessary to shave a larger surface area than the immediate surgical site. He may fear that the surgical incision will be as large as the area shaved.

Pediatric Considerations

Clipping is not used for young children. Adolescents who have more and longer body hair may have clipping performed.

Nasogastric Tube Insertion, Placement, and Anchoring

Insertion of a nasogastric tube involves placing a pliable plastic tube through the client's nasopharynx into the stomach. The tube has a hollow lumen that allows both the removal of gastric secretions from and the introduction of solutions into the stomach.

Potential Nursing Diagnoses

Clients requiring nasogastric tube insertion, placement, and anchoring may have one or more of the following nursing diagnoses:

Alteration in comfort related to nasogastric tube placement and abdominal distention

Potential fluid volume deficit related to prolonged vomiting

Anxiety related to insertion of nasogastric tube

Equipment

Nasogastric tube (14 or 16 gauge French)
Water-soluble lubricating jelly
Stethoscope
Tongue blade
Flashlight
Soft bulb syringe or cone tip (30-50 ml) syringe
Hypoallergenic tape 2.5 cm (1-inch) wide
Safety pin and rubber band
Clamp, drainage bag, or suction machine
Bath towel
Emesis basin with ice (optional)

Glass of water with straw
Facial tissues

Steps	Rationale
Tube Insertion	
1. Explain the procedure fully to client, as well as purpose of nasogastric decompression.	Procedure is easier to complete with client's full cooperation.
2. Wash hands.	Reduces transfer of microorganisms.
3. Assemble all equipment at bedside.	Organized procedure can be performed in a timely fashion, limiting client's discomfort.
4. If nasogastric tube is too pliable, place it in emesis basin and cover with ice.	Stiffens tube for easier insertion.
5. Assist client to high Fowler position with pillows behind head and shoulders.	Promotes client's ability to swallow.
6. Place bath towel over client's chest. Keep facial tissues within client's reach.	Prevents soiling of client's gown. Insertion of tube through nasal passages may cause tearing.
7. Stand on right side of bed if you are right handed (or on left side if left-handed).	Allows easier manipulating of tubing.
8. Instruct client to relax and breathe normally while occluding one naris. Then repeat procedure for other naris. Select one with greater air flow.	Tube passes more easily through naris that is more patent.

Steps	Rationale
9. Estimate distance to insert tube by placing tip of tube at client's nose and extending tube to tip of earlobe and down to xiphoid process (at base of sternum). (Fig. 146)	Tube should extend from naris to stomach (distance varying for each client).
10. Curve 10-15 cm (4-6 inches) of tube tightly around your index finger and then release.	Aids tube insertion.
11. Lubricate 7.5-10 cm (3-4 inches) of tube with water-soluble jelly.	Minimizes friction against nasal mucosa. (Water-soluble lubricant cannot cause aspiration pneumonia if it accidentally enters lungs as lipid-soluble agent can.)
12. Instruct client to initially extend neck. Insert tube slowly through naris with curved end pointing downward.	Facilitates initial passage of tube through naris and maintains clear airway for open naris.

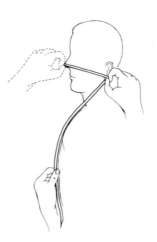

Fig. 146

Steps	Rationale
13. Continue to pass tube along floor of nasal passage. When resistance is felt, apply gentle downward pressure to advance tube. (Do not force tube past resistance.)	Minimizes discomfort of tube rubbing against upper nasal turbinates. Resistance is created by posterior nasopharynx.
14. If you meet resistance, withdraw tube and relubricate. Insert it in other naris.	Forcing against resistance can cause trauma to mucosa.
15. Stop tube advancement briefly. Allow client to relax. Provide tissues. Explain that next step requires client to swallow.	Relieves client's anxiety. Tearing is a natural response to mucosal irritation.
16. With tube just above oropharynx, instruct client to tilt head forward and dry swallow or suck in air through straw. Advance tube 2.5-5 cm (1-2 inches) with each swallow. If client has trouble swallowing and can take fluids, offer glass of water. Advance tube with each swallow of water.	Flexed position closes off upper airway to trachea and opens esophagus. Swallowing aids entrance of tube into esophagus; swallowing water reduces gagging.
17. If client begins to cough, gag, or choke, stop tube advancement momentarily. Have client breathe easily. Offer another sip of water.	Tube may be entering larynx and initiating cough reflex. Gagging can be eased by swallowing water.
18. Withdraw tube slightly if client continues coughing.	Tube entering larynx will obstruct airway.
19. If gagging continues, check back of pharynx with tongue blade and flashlight.	Tube may be sliding in back of throat.

Steps	Rationale
20. Once client is at ease, continue to advance tube desired distance.	Tip of tube should be within stomach to decompress properly.

Checking Tube Placement

1. Attach a syringe to end of nasogastric tube. Place diaphragm of stethoscope over upper left quadrant of client's abdomen just below costal margin. Inject 10-20 ml of air while auscultating abdomen. (Fig. 147)	Air entering stomach creates "whooshing" sound and confirms tube placement. Absence of sound indicates tip of tube is still in esophagus.
2. Aspirate gently to obtain gastric contents.	Another effective means for confirming tube placement. If tip is not in stomach, contents cannot be aspirated.
3. If tube is not in stomach, advance another 2.5-5 cm (1-2 inches) and again check position.	Tube must be in stomach to provide adequate decompression.

Anchoring Tube

1. Once tube is properly inserted, either clamp or connect end to drainage bag or suction machine.	Clients going to surgery often will have tube clamped. Drainage bag provides for gravity drainage. Intermittent

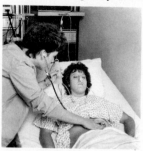

Fig. 147

Steps	Rationale
	suction is most effective in providing decompression.
2. Tape tube to client's nose, avoiding pressure on naris. Take 10 cm (4-inch) piece of tape. Split one end lengthwise 5 cm (2 inches). Place other end over bridge of nose. Wrap 1.3 cm (½-inch) strips around tube as it exits nose. (Fig. 148)	Prevents tissue necrosis.
3. Fasten end of nasogastric tube to client's gown by looping a ruber band around tube in slip knot and pinning rubber band	Reduces traction on naris during movement of tube.

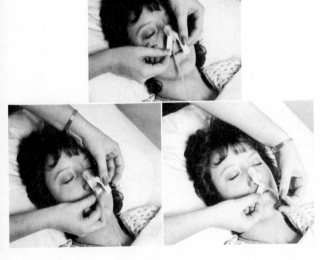

Fig. 148

Steps	Rationale
to gown. (Allow slack for movement.)	
4. Wash hands.	Reduces transfer of microorganisms.
5. Record insertion procedure in nurse's notes. Mention specifically type of tube inserted, tube placement, drainage return, and client's tolerance.	Timely recording accurately documents performance of procedure.

Nurse Alert

Nasogastric tube placement can be confirmed accurately only by x-ray visualization and must be reassessed after the client's position changes or if severe coughing or vomiting develops. Verification determines that the tube is not displaced from the stomach into the airway.

Client Teaching

Preprocedure instruction in relaxation and deep breathing exercises can help reduce client anxiety and promote cooperation during tube insertion.

Pediatric Considerations

Nasogastric tubes may be placed in infants or small children through either the mouth or the nares. The size of the tube varies with the size of the child and the viscosity of any solution being introduced (infants, 5 to 8 Fr; children, 10 to 14 Fr). Measurement is from (a) the bridge of the nose to the umbilicus or (b) the tip of the nose to the earlobe and then to the tip of the xiphoid process.

Geriatric Considerations

With aging there is a reduction in the amount of secretions produced by the stomach and intestinal tract.

Irrigating a Nasogastric Tube

A nasogastric tube is irrigated to maintain patency. If the distal tip of the tube rests against the stomach wall or if the tube becomes occluded with secretions, it must be irrigated. Obstruction of the tube can result in abdominal distention and possible vomiting. Nasogastric tube irrigations are routinely ordered when intermittent gastric suction is ordered.

Potential Nursing Diagnoses

Clients requiring nasogastric tube irrigation may have one or more of the following nursing diagnoses:

Alteration in comfort related to abdominal distention or nausea

Potential fluid volume deficit related to nasogastric tube drainage

Potential alteration in nasal mucosa related to presence of nasogastric tube

Equipment

Soft or small bulb syringe or GU syringe
Normal saline, 30 ml
Emesis basin or irrigation tray
Towel
Facial tissues

Steps	Rationale
1. Wash hands.	Reduces transmission of microorganisms.
2. Check tube placement.	Prevents accidental entrance of irrigating solution into lungs.
▪ Attach syringe to end of nasogastric tube. Place diaphragm of stethoscope over upper left quadrant of client's abdomen just below costal margin. Inject 10-20 ml of air while auscultating abdomen.	Air entering stomach creates "whooshing" sound and confirms tube placement. Absence of sound indicates that tip of tube is still in esophagus.
▪ Aspirate gently to obtain gastric contents.	If tip is not in stomach, contents cannot be aspirated.
▪ If tube is not in stomach, advance another 2.5-5 cm (1-2 inches) and check position.	Tubing must be in stomach to provide adequate decompression.
3. Draw up 30 ml of normal saline into bulb syringe.	Isotonic solution maintains osmotic pressure and minimizes loss of electrolytes from stomach.
4. Kink or clamp off tube proximal to connection site of drainage or suction apparatus. Disconnect suction tube and lay end on towel.	Prevents backflow of secretions and soiling of client's gown and bed linen.
5. Insert tip of irrigating syringe into end of nasogastric tube. Release clamp or kink in tube. Holding syringe with tip toward floor, inject saline slowly but evenly. (Do not force.)	Position of syringe prevents introduction of air into tubing. Air can cause distention. Fluid introduced under pressure can cause trauma.
6. If resistance occurs, check for kinks in tubing. Turn client on his side. Re-	Buildup of secretions will cause abdominal distention.

Steps	Rationale
peated resistance should be reported to physician.	
7. After instilling saline, immediately aspirate to withdraw fluid. Measure volume returned.	Stomach should remain empty. Fluid in stomach is measured as intake.
8. Reconnect nasogastric tube to drainage or suction. (If flow does not return, irrigation may be repeated.)	Reestablishes means of collecting drainage.
9. Record irrigation procedure in nurse's notes. Mention specifically amount of normal saline instilled, amount and type of drainage returned, and client's tolerance.	Documents performance of procedure.

Nurse Alert

If a nasogastric tube continues to drain improperly after irrigation, the nurse must reposition it by advancing or withdrawing it slightly. Changes in the client's position or severe coughing or vomiting require reassessment of tube placement.

Client Teaching

Instruct the client to notify nursing personnel if the nasogastric tube becomes displaced or he feels nauseated. Nausea may be associated with abdominal distention due to improper draining of the tube. Irrigation of the tube may improve drainage and relieve the nausea.

Pediatric Considerations

Children are vulnerable to fluid and electrolyte imbalances associated with nasogastric suctioning. Therefore a meticulously accurate record of drainage and irrigating solution is essential.

For irrigation an electrolyte solution is used to prevent further body depletion.

Geriatric Considerations

The older adult is vulnerable to fluid and electrolyte imbalances associated with nasogastric suctioning. Therefore accurate recording of drainage and irrigating solution is essential.

Clients with a nasogastric tube are NPO. An elderly person's oral mucosa can become dry and inflamed without thorough hygiene. Thus during nasogastric suctioning it is essential to keep the mucosa well hydrated.

Discontinuing a Nasogastric Tube

Discontinuing a nasogastric tube is done when the client no longer needs gastric decompression, feeding, or lavage. Discontinuation of the nasogastric tube requires a physician's order.

Potential Nursing Diagnoses

Clients who require discontinuation of a nasogastric tube may have either or both of the following nursing diagnoses:

Alteration in comfort related to presence of nasogastric tube

Alteration in nasal or oral mucous membrane related to nasogastric tube

Equipment

Facial tissue
Towel
Emesis basin
Toothbrush or sponge applicators for mouth care

Steps	Rationale
1. Wash hands.	Reduces transfer of microorganisms.
2. Place towel under client's chin.	Prevents contamination of bed or gown from gastric secretions.

383

Steps	Rationale
3. Turn off suction and disconnect nasogastric tube from drainage bag. Remove tape from bridge of nose and remove pin from gown.	Tube should be free of connection when removed.
4. Explain procedure to client, reassuring him that removal is less distressing than insertion.	Minimizes client's anxiety.
5. Hand client a facial tissue. Instruct him to take a deep breath and hold.	Airway may be temporarily obstructed during removal of tube. NOTE: Some clients may experience paroxysms of coughing during procedure.
6. Pull tube steadily and smoothly as client is holding his breath. (Do not pull too slowly or too rapidly.)	Reduces trauma to mucosa and minimizes client discomfort.
7. Dispose of tube and drainage equipment and wash hands.	Reduces transfer of microorganisms.
8. Clean client's nares and provide mouth care.	Promotes comfort. Nares often become excoriated.
9. Record procedure in nurse's notes. Mention specifically tube removal, final volume of secretions collected in drainage system, and client's response.	Timely recording accurately documents procedure.

Nurse Alert

After discontinuing a nasogastric tube the nurse should observe the client for abdominal distention, nausea, or vomiting. Any of these signs or symptoms could indicate the need for reinserting the tube.

Inserting a Dobhoff Tube

The Dobhoff tube is a small-bore, soft, flexible tube manufactured of Silastic and weighted with mercury to facilitate its passage. Due to its flexibility, it requires a small nylon guidewire to provide rigidity. A Dobhoff tube is inserted when the client requires long-term nasogastric feeding. Because it is soft and flexible, the risk of trauma to the nasal mucosa is reduced. Clients also report less gagging with the small-bore tube.

Potential Nursing Diagnoses

Clients requiring a Dobhoff tube may have one or more of the following nursing diagnoses:

Potential alterations in self-concept related to invasive feeding tube

Alterations in comfort related to feeding tube

Alterations in nutrition: less than body requirements

Equipment

Dobhoff tube
Guidewire
Water-soluble lubricant
Tape
Tincture of benzoin

Glass of water and straw
Towel
Tongue blade
Facial tissues

Steps	Rationale
1. Wash hands.	Reduces transmission of microorganisms.
2. Explain procedure to client.	Promotes cooperation at time of tube insertion and helps relieve anxiety.
3. Assemble all equipment at bedside.	Facilitates performance of procedure, thus limiting client's discomfort.
4. Assist client to a sitting or high Fowler position with neck hyperextended.	Facilitates passage of tube into client's stomach.
5. Place bath towel over client's chest. Keep facial tissues within reach.	Prevents soiling of client's gown. Insertion of tube through nasal passages may cause tearing.
6. Stand on right side of bed if right handed.	Allows easier manipulation of tubing.
7. Instruct client to relax and breathe normally while occluding one naris. Then repeat procedure for other naris. Select one with greater air flow.	Tube passes more easily through naris that is more patent.
8. Determine length of tube to be inserted: ■ Measure distance from tip of nose to earlobe to xyphoid process (of sternum).	Prevents improper positioning of tube.
9. Inspect tube for sharp edges at distal end or closed or clogged outlet holes.	Prevents intubation with a defective tube.
10. Insert guidewire into tube.	Provides rigidity and eases passage into stomach.

Steps	Rationale
11. Lubricate 7.5-10 cm (3-4 inches) of tube with water-soluble lubricant.	Decreases trauma to nasal turbinates while tube is being inserted. Water-soluble lubricant is used. A lipid-soluble lubricant would increase risk of lipid aspiration.
12. Instruct client to extend his neck. Insert tube slowly through naris.	Facilitates initial passage of tube through naris and maintains clear airway for open naris.
13. Continue inserting tube, projecting it gently downward and back toward pharynx. *Do not force*.	Follow natural anatomic contours. This will facilitate passage of the tube.
14. Encourage client to swallow as tube is advanced. NOTE: Gagging is minimal with Dobhoff tube.	Facilitates passage of tube past oropharynx.
15. If client begins to cough or choke, stop tube advancement.	Tube may be entering larynx and initiating cough reflex.
16. Aspirate gastric contents by attaching syringe to distal portion of tube and gently drawing.	Verifies correct placement of tube in client's stomach. NOTE: Some agencies may verify placement by obtaining abdominal x-ray projection.
17. Secure tube with tape and anchor it to client's gown (Skill 9-1).	Prevents extubation and maintains correct positioning.
18. Wash hands.	Reduces transmission of microorganisms.
19. Record procedure in nurse's notes.	Documents insertion, placement, and position of tube.

Nurse Alert

Because the Dobhoff tube is small bore, the nurse cannot verify its placement by injecting air and auscultating at the client's abdomen. The auscultation method can be used only for large-bore tubes. Verification is achieved by aspirating gastric contents or abdominal x-ray.

Client Teaching

Preprocedure education reduces the client's anxiety and increases his cooperation.

Pediatric Considerations

Infants or young children will likely need restraining during tube insertion. Infants are obligatory nose breathers, and insertion of a feeding tube through the mouth causes less distress as well as helps promote normal sucking.

DRESSINGS, BINDERS, AND BANDAGES

Changing a Dry Dressing

A dry dressing protects wounds with minimal drainage against microorganism contamination. The dressing can be simply a gauze pad that does not adhere to wound tissues and causes very little irritation. Or it can be a Telfa pad that, likewise, does not adhere to the incision or wound opening but allows drainage through the nonadherent surface to the softened gauze beneath.

As long as an incision or wound remains open, the application of a dry dressing requires sterile technique.

Potential Nursing Diagnoses

Clients who require dry dressings may have one or more of the following nursing diagnoses:

Impairment of skin integrity related to surgical incision or traumatic wound.

Alteration in comfort related to incisional wound

Impaired mobility related to incisional pain

Equipment

Sterile dressing set or individual supplies of following:
Sterile gloves
Dressing set (scissors and forceps)
Gauze dressings and pads
Basin for antiseptic or cleaning solution
Antiseptic ointment (optional)
Cleaning solution prescribed by physician
Normal saline or water

Disposable gloves
Tape, ties, or bandage as needed
Waterproof bag for disposal
Extra gauze dressings and Surgipads or ABD pads.
Bath blanket
Acetone (optional)

Steps	Rationale
1. Explain procedure to client by describing steps of wound care.	Relieves client anxiety and promotes understanding of healing process.
2. Assemble all necessary supplies at bedside table (do not yet open supplies).	Prevents chances of break in sterile technique by accidental omission of needed supply.
3. Take disposable bag and make cuff at top. Place bag within reach of your work area.	Prevents accidental contamination of top of outer bag surface. You should not reach across sterile field to dispose of soiled dressing.
4. Close room or cubicle curtains or arrange partition around bed. Close any open windows.	Provides client privacy and reduces air currents that may transmit microorganisms.
5. Assist client to comfortable position and drape him with bath blanket to expose only wound site. Instruct client not to touch wound area or sterile supplies.	Sudden movement by client during dressing change can cause contamination of wound or supplies. Draping provides access to wound and minimizes unnecessary exposure.
6. Wash hands thoroughly.	Removes microorganisms resident on skin surface and reduces transmission of pathogens to exposed tissues.
7. Don clean disposable gloves and remove tape, ties, or bandage.	Gloves prevent transmission of infectious organisms from soiled dressings to your hands.

Steps	Rationale
8. Remove tape by loosening end and pulling gently, parallel to skin and toward dressing. (If adhesive remains on skin, it may be removed with acetone.)	Reduces tension against suture line or wound edges.
9. With your gloved hand or forceps, lift dressings off, keeping soiled undersurface away from client's sight. NOTE: If drains are present, remove only a layer at a time.	Appearance of drainage may upset client emotionally. Cautious removal of dressings prevents accidental withdrawal of drain.
10. If dressing sticks to wound, loosen it by applying sterile saline or water.	Prevents disruption of epidermal surface.
11. Observe character and amount of drainage on dressings.	Provides estimate of drainage lost and assessment of wound's condition.
12. Dispose of soiled dressings in trash bag, avoiding contamination of bag's outer surface. Remove disposable gloves by pulling them inside out. Dispose of them properly.	Procedures reduce transmission of microorganisms to other persons.
13. Open sterile dressing tray or individually wrapped sterile supplies. Place on bedside table or at client's side on bed. Dressings, scissors, and forceps should remain in sterile tray or can be placed on open sterile drape used as a sterile field. Open bottle	Sterile dressings and supplies remain sterile while on or within a sterile surface. Preparation of all supplies prevents break in technique during actual dressing change.

Steps	Rationale
or packet of antiseptic solution and pour it into sterile basin or over sterile gauze. (Fig. 149)	
14. If sterile drape or gauze packages become wet from antiseptic solution, repeat preparation of supplies.	Fluids move through material by capillary action. Microorganisms travel from unsterile environment on table top or bed linen through dressing package to dressing itself.
15. Don sterile gloves. (Fig. 150)	Allows you to handle sterile dressings, instruments, and solutions without contaminating them.
16. Inspect wound. Note its condition, placement of drain, integrity of suture or skin closure, and character of drainage. (Palpate wound, if necessary, with portion of nondominant hand that will not touch sterile supplies.) (Fig. 151)	Determines state of wound healing. (Contact with skin surface or drainage contaminates glove.)

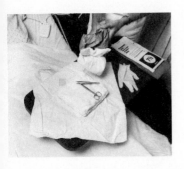

Fig. 149

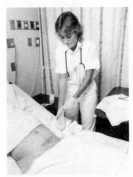

Fig. 150

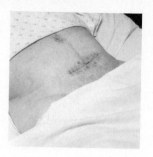

Fig. 151

Steps	Rationale
17. Clean wound with prescribed antiseptic solution or normal saline. Grasp gauze moistened in solution with forceps. Use separate gauze for each cleaning stroke. Clean from least contaminated to most contaminated area. Move in progressive strokes away from incision line or wound edges.	Use of forceps prevents contamination of gloved fingers. Direction of cleaning strokes prevents introduction of organisms into wound.
18. Use fresh gauze to dry wound or incision line. Swab in same manner as described in Step 17.	Reduces moisture at wound site, which eventually could harbor microorganisms.
19. Apply antiseptic ointment (if ordered), using same technique as for cleaning. Do not apply over drainage site.	Application directly to dressing or drainage site can occlude drainage.
20. Apply dry sterile dressings to incision or wound site.	
▪ Apply dressings one at a time. (Fig. 152)	Prevents application of large bulky dressings that may impair client's movement and ensures proper coverage of entire wound.

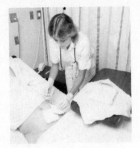

Fig. 152

Steps	Rationale
▪ Apply loose woven gauze (4 × 4) or Telfa as contact layer.	Promotes proper absorption of drainage.
▪ If a drain is present, take scissors and cut 4 × 4 gauze square to fit around it.	Dressing around drain secures its placement and absorbs drainage.
▪ Apply second layer of gauze as an absorbent layer.	
▪ Apply thicker woven Surgipad or ABD pad. (Blue line down middle of pad marks outside surface.) (Fig. 153)	Protects wound from entrance of microorganisms.

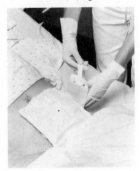

Fig. 153

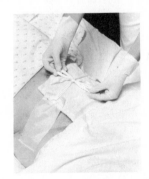

Fig. 154

Steps	Rationale
21. Use tape over dressing or secure with Montgomery ties, bandage, or binder. (Fig. 154)	Provides support to wound and ensures complete coverage with minimized exposure to microorganisms.
22. Remove gloves and dispose of them properly in container.	Reduces transmission of microorganisms.
23. Dispose of all supplies and help client return to comfortable position.	Clean environment enhances client comfort.
24. Wash hands.	Reduces microorganism transmission.
25. Record in nurse's notes observations of wound, dressing, and drainage. Document dressing change, including statement of client's response.	Accurate timely documentation notifies personnel of any changes in wound condition and status of client.

Nurse Alert

When removing or positioning the dressing, take care not to dislodge or pull on a drain. If the wound is dry and intact, healing may be optimized by exposing it to air. Contact the physician for an order to discontinue wound dressing.

Client Teaching

Clients often go home with a simple dry dressing in place. They, or their family, must be instructed in handwashing techniques, wound cleaning, and proper disposal of soiled dressings. It is not necessary to use sterile technique.

Pediatric Considerations

When a dressing is absolutely necessary in an infant or young child, the nurse should incorporate diversional activities into her care plan so the chances of the child's displacing the dressing will be minimized.

Geriatric Considerations

An elderly client's skin is normally inelastic and thin. Use special care, therefore, when removing tape.

Changing a Wet-to-Dry Dressing

A wet-to-dry dressing is the treatment of choice for wounds requiring debridement. The wet portion of the dressing effectively cleans an infected and necrotic wound. The moist gauze directly absorbs all exudate and wound debris. The dry outer layer helps pull moisture from the wound into the dressing by capillary action.

Potential Nursing Diagnoses

Clients who require a wet-to-dry dressing may have one or more of the following nursing diagnoses:

Impaired skin integrity related to wound infection
Potential for injury related to open wound
Alteration in comfort related to wound drainage
Disturbance in self-concept related to wound drainage

Equipment

A sterile dressing set or individual supplies of following:
Sterile gloves
Sterile scissors and forceps
Sterile drape (optional)
Gauze dressings and fine-mesh 4 × 4 gauze pads
Basin for antiseptic or cleaning solution
Antiseptic ointment (optional)
Cleaning solution prescribed by physician
Normal saline or water
Disposable gloves
Tape, ties, or bandage as needed

Waterproof bag for disposal
Extra gauze dressings and Surgipads or ABD pads.
Bath blanket
Acetone (optional)
Waterproof pad

Steps	Rationale
1. Explain procedure to client by describing steps of wound care.	Relieves client's anxiety and promotes understanding of healing process.
2. Assemble all necessary supplies at bedside table (do not yet open supplies).	Prevents chances of break in sterile technique by accidental omission of a needed supply.
3. Take disposable bag and make cuff at top. Place bag within reach of your work area.	Cuff prevents accidental contamination of top of outer bag surface. You should not reach across sterile field to dispose of soiled dressing.
4. Close room or cubicle curtains or arrange partition around bed. Close any open windows.	Provides client privacy and reduces air currents that may transmit microorganisms.
5. Assist client to comfortable position and drape him with bath blanket to expose only wound site. Instruct client not to touch wound area or sterile supplies.	Sudden movement by client during dressing change can cause contamination of wound or supplies. Draping provides access to wound and minimizes unnecessary exposure.
6. Wash hands thoroughly.	Removes microorganisms resident on skin surface and reduces transmission of pathogens to exposed tissues.
7. Place waterproof pad under client.	Prevents soiling of bed linen.
8. Don clean disposable gloves and remove tape, ties, or bandage.	Gloves prevent transmission of infectious organisms from soiled dressings to your hands.

Steps	Rationale
9. Remove tape by loosening end and pulling gently, parallel to skin and toward dressing. (If adhesive remains on skin, it may be removed with acetone.)	Reduces tension against suture line or wound edges.
10. With gloved hand or forceps, lift dressings off, keeping soiled undersurface away from client's sight. NOTE: If drains are present, remove only a layer at a time.	Appearance of drainage may upset client emotionally. Cautious removal of dressings prevents accidental withdrawal of drain.
11. If dressing adheres to underlying tissues, do not moisten it. Gently free the dressing from dried exudate. Warn client about pulling and possible discomfort.	Wet-to-dry dressing is designed to clean contaminated or infected wounds by debridement of necrotic tissue and exudate.
12. Observe character and amount of drainage on dressing.	Provides estimate of drainage lost and assessment of wound condition.
13. Dispose of soiled dressings in appropriate container, avoiding contamination of outer surface of container. Remove disposable gloves by pulling them inside out. Dispose of them properly.	Reduces transmission of microorganisms to other persons.
14. Prepare sterile dressing supplies. Pour the prescribed solution into a sterile basin and add fine-mesh gauze.	Contact layer of gauze must be totally moistened to increase dressing's absorptive abilities.

Steps	Rationale
15. Don sterile gloves.	Allows you to handle sterile dressings, instruments, and solutions without contaminating them with microorganisms.
16. Inspect wound. Note its condition, placement of drain, integrity of sutures or skin closure, and character of drainage. (Palpate wound, if necessary, with portion of your nondominant hand that will not be touching sterile supplies.)	Determines state of wound healing. (Contact with skin surface or drainage contaminates glove.)
17. Clean wound with prescribed antiseptic solution or normal saline. Grasp gauze moistened in solution with forceps. Use separate gauze square for each cleaning stroke. Clean from least contaminated to most contaminated area. Move in progressive strokes away from incision line or wound edges.	Use of forceps prevents contamination of your gloved fingers. Direction of cleaning prevents introduction of organisms into wound.
18. Apply moist fine-mesh gauze directly on wound surface. If wound is deep, gently pack it by first picking up end of gauze with forceps. Gradually feed gauze into wound so all surfaces of wound are in contact with moist gauze. (Figs. 155 and 156)	Moist gauze absorbs drainage and adheres to debris. Pack gauze so it is evenly distributed within wound bed.
19. Apply dry sterile gauze (4 × 4) over wet gauze.	Dry layer serves as absorbent layer to pull moisture from wound surface.

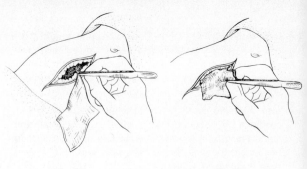

Fig. 155   Fig. 156

Steps	Rationale
20. Cover with gauze, Surgipad, or ABD pad.	Gauze or pad protects wound from entrance of microorganisms.
21. Apply tape over dressing or secure with Montgomery ties, bandage, or binder.	Provides support to wound and ensures complete coverage of wound to minimize exposure to microorganisms.
22. Assist client to comfortable position.	Enhances client's sense of well-being.
23. Wash hands.	Reduces transmission of microorganisms.
24. Record in nurse's notes observations of wound, dressing, drainage, and client's response.	Accurate and timely documentation notifies personnel of any changes in wound condition and status of client.

Nurse Alert

Removal of the old dressing and reapplication of a new wet-to-dry dressing may cause the client pain. The nurse should administer an analgesic and time the dressing change to coincide with the drug's peak effect.

Client Teaching

A client is not usually discharged home while a wet-to-dry dressing is still required. He can be taught wound care in anticipation of use of a dry dressing at home.

Pediatric Considerations

It may be necessary to reinforce a wet-to-dry dressing with a gauze roll to prevent its accidental removal by an active toddler. Whenever possible, reinforce the dressing rather than restrain the child.

Geriatric Considerations

An elderly client's skin is normally thin and inelastic. Use special care, therefore, when removing tape.

Wound Irrigation

The purpose of wound irrigation is to remove exudate and debris from slow-healing wounds. It requires sterile technique and is particularly useful for open deep wounds, when access to all wound surfaces is limited. Wound irrigation can deliver heat to an affected area to promote healing or facilitate the application of local medications.

Potential Nursing Diagnoses

Clients who require wound irrigation may have one or more of the following nursing diagnoses:

Impairment of skin integrity related to wound infection

Alteration in comfort related to wound drainage or inflammation

Disturbance in self-concept related to wound drainage

Equipment

Sterile basin

Irrigating solution (200-500 ml as ordered) warmed to body temperature (32°-37° C or 90°-98.6° F)

Sterile irrigating syringe (sterile red rubber catheter as an attachment for deep wounds with small openings)

Clean basin to receive solution

Sterile dressing tray and supplies for dressing change

Waterproof pad

Lubricating jelly and tongue blade (optional)

Steps	Rationale
1. Explain procedure to client. Describe sensations to be felt during irrigation	Client's anxiety will be reduced through awareness of what procedure involves and sensations to be expected.
2. Assemble supplies at bedside.	Prevents break in procedure.
3. Position client so irrigating solution will flow from upper end of wound into basin held below wound. (Fig. 157)	Fluid flows by gravity from least to most contaminated area.
4. Place waterproof pad under client.	Prevents soiling of bed linen.
5. Wash hands.	Reduces microorganism transmission.
6. Don clean disposable gloves and remove tape, ties, or bandage.	Gloves prevent transmission of infectious organisms from soiled dressings to your hands.
7. Remove tape by loosening end and pulling gently, parallel with skin and toward dressing. (If adhesive remains on the skin, it may be removed with acetone.)	Reduces tension against suture line or wound edges.

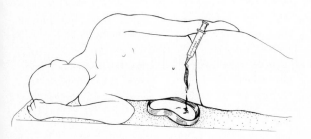

Fig. 157

Steps	Rationale
8. With your gloved hand or forceps, lift dressings off, keeping soiled undersurface away from client's sight. Remove one dressing layer at a time.	Appearance of drainage may upset client emotionally. Cautious removal of dressings prevents accidental withdrawal of drain.
9. If dressing sticks to wound, loosen it by applying sterile saline or water.	Prevents disruption of epidermal surface.
10. Observe character and amount of drainage on dressings.	Provides estimate of drainage lost and assessment of wound's condition.
11. Dispose of soiled dressings in proper receptacle, avoiding contamination of receptacle's outer surface. Remove disposable gloves by pulling them inside out. Dispose of them properly.	Reduces transmission of microorganisms to other persons.
12. Prepare sterile supplies. Open basin and pour in solution (volume varies depending on size of wound and extent of drainage). Open syringe. Prepare dressing tray. Don sterile gloves.	Prevents introduction of microorganisms into wound.
13. Place clean basin against client's skin below incision or wound site.	Collects contaminated irrigating solution.
14. Draw up some solution into syringe. While holding syringe tip just above top of wound, irrigate slowly but continuously with enough force to flush away drainage and debris. Avoid sudden spurts or splashing of fluid. Irrigate pockets in wound.	Irrigation mechanically removes drainage and debris. Pockets or depressions in wound bed can easily trap debris.

Steps	Rationale
15. Continue irrigating until solution draining into basin is clear.	Ensures that all debris has been removed.
16. With sterile gauze, dry off wound edges. Clean from least contaminated to most contaminated area. Move in progressive strokes away from incision line or wound edges.	Removes excess moisture, which can serve as medium for microorganism growth or as irritant to skin.
17. Apply sterile dressing.	Sterile dressing prevents infection and promotes wound healing.
18. Assist client to comfortable position.	Promotes client comfort.
19. Dispose of equipment and wash hands.	Controls transfer of microorganisms.
20. Record in nurse's notes volume and type of solution, character of drainage, appearance of wound, and client's response.	Timely recording provides accurate documentation of therapy and progress of wound healing.

Nurse Alert

If drains are present, remove only one layer of dressing at a time so accidental withdrawal of a drain does not occur. Do not forcibly introduce irrigant into a wound pocket that is not visible. You could damage tissue.

Client Teaching

The client is not usually discharged home when irrigations are still necessary. However, instruct him regarding the procedure for wound irrigations so he can monitor the progress of his healing. In addition, early instruction helps him and his family prepare for discharge and any necessary home care.

Pediatric Considerations

If a child is unable to remain still during the procedure, it may be helpful for another nurse or the parent to use diversional activites such as reading, singing, or storytelling. Cautious use of restraints may be necessary.

Ear Irrigation

Irrigation of the auditory canal is performed to remove cerumen or a foreign object or to apply heat. The irrigating solution should be sterile to prevent transmission of microorganisms in the event of tympanic membrane rupture. The solution must be room temperature so it does not cause nausea or vertigo (severe dizziness). At home the client or family can be instructed in proper cleaning of the ear to reduce the need for further irrigation.

Potential Nursing Diagnoses

Clients who require irrigation of the auditory canal may have one or more of the following nursing diagnoses:

Potential for injury related to presence of foreign body in auditory canal

Potential for sensory-perceptual alteration: auditory, related to obstruction of ear canal

Alteration in comfort related to inflammation of auditory canal

Equipment

Prescribed irrigating solution; volume depends on purpose: 200-500 ml at 37° C (98.6° F)

Sterile basin for solution

Soft or small bulb syringe

Curved emesis basin

Moisture-proof towel or pad

Cotton-tip applicators

Bath thermometer

Cotton balls

Steps	Rationale
1. Wash hands.	Reduces transmission of microorganisms.
2. Explain steps of procedure and warn client about sensations that might be experienced.	Relieves client's anxiety.
3. Assist client to either a side-lying or a sitting position with head tilted toward affected ear. Position emesis basin under ear. (Client may help hold basin.)	Irrigating solution will flow from auditory canal into basin.
4. Place towel over client's shoulder just under ear and emesis basin.	Prevents soiling of gown and bed linen.
5. Inspect auditory canal for any accumulation of cerumen or debris. Remove with cotton applicator and solution.	Prevents reentrance of debris into canal during irrigation.
6. Check irrigating solution for proper temperature. Fill bulb syringe with appropriate volume.	Solution at body temperature minimizes onset of dizziness and discomfort.
7. Straighten auditory canal for introduction of solution. In infants, pull auricle (or pinna) down and back. In adults, pull auricle up and back.	Facilitates entrance and flow of irrigating solution.
8. With tip of syringe just above canal, irrigate gently by creating steady flow of solution against roof of canal.	Occlusion of canal with syringe causes pressure against tympanic membrane during irrigation. Flow of solution drains safely out of canal while loosening debris.

Steps	Rationale
9. Continue irrigation until all debris has been removed or all solution has been used.	Purpose of irrigation may be to clean canal, instill antiseptics, or provide local heat.
10. Assess client for onset of dizziness or nausea. Onset of symptoms may require temporary cessation of procedure.	Irritation of semicircular canals may cause dizziness and nausea.
11. Dry off auricle and apply cotton ball to auditory meatus.	Drying promotes client's comfort. Cotton ball collects excess drainage.
12. Position client on side of affected ear for 10 minutes.	Remaining solution in auditory canal will drain out.
13. Remove equipment and wash hands.	Controls transfer of microorganisms.
14. Return to client to assess character and amount of drainage and determine his level of comfort.	Enables you to evaluate client's tolerance of procedure.
15. Record in nurse's notes client's response to irrigation and note type, temperature, and volume of solution used and character of drainage.	Timely recording provides accurate documentation of client's response to procedure.
16. Return to client after 10 minutes to remove cotton ball and reassess drainage. Client may resume normal level of activity.	Increase in drainage or onset of pain may indicate injury to tympanic membrane.

Nurse Alert

Although the external auditory canal is not sterile, nevertheless you should use sterile drops and solutions in case the tympanic membrane (eardrum) is ruptured. Entrance of nonsterile solutions into the middle ear could result in infection. Never occlude the external auditory canal with the syringe. Forceful delivery of solution can damage the tympanic membrane.

Client Teaching

Family members as well as the client should be instructed not to force medication into an occluded auditory canal. Instilling medication or solution under pressure can injure the eardrum.

Pediatric Considerations

The auditory canal of infants and young children is straightened by grasping the pinna and pulling it gently downward and backward. Failure to straighten the canal properly may prevent medicinal solutions from reaching the deeper external ear structures.

Geriatric Considerations

The skin lining the auditory canal of an elderly person often becomes dry, flaky, and irritated. It is thus very important to be gentle when performing irrigations or cleanings of the ear in older clients.

Eye Irrigation

Eye irrigation is performed to relieve local inflammation of the conjunctiva, apply antiseptic solution, or flush out exudate or caustic or irritating solutions. It is a procedure commonly used in emergency situations when a foreign object or some other substance has entered the eye. Many of the principles used in this procedure are the same as in Skill 4-9.

Potential Nursing Diagnoses

Clients who require eye irrigation may have one or more of the following nursing diagnoses:

Sensory alteration: visual, related to inflammation and/or injury

Alteration in comfort related to corneal or conjunctival injury

Anxiety related to loss of vision

Equipment

Prescribed irrigating solution; volume varies: 30-180 ml at 37° C (98.6° F) (For chemical flushing: tap water in volume to provide continuous irrigation over 15 minutes)

Sterile basin for solution

Curved emesis basin

Waterproof pad or towel

Cotton balls

Soft bulb syringe or eye dropper

Disposable gloves (optional)

Steps	Rationale
1. Explain procedure fully to client. Explain that he will be allowed to close eye periodically and that no object will touch eye.	Relieves client's anxiety and improves his ability to cooperate.
2. Assist client to lying position on side of affected eye. Turn his head toward affected eye.	Irrigating solution will flow from inner to outer canthus and into collecting basin.
3. Wash your hands.	Reduces number of microorganisms on skin surface.
4. Don disposable gloves (if client's eye is infected).	Prevents exposure of your hands to pathogens.
5. Place waterproof pad under client's face.	Prevents soiling of bed linen.
6. With cotton ball moistened in prescribed solution (or normal saline), gently clean lid margins and eyelashes. Clean from inner to outer canthus.	Minimizes transfer of debris from lids or lashes into eye during irrigation. Cleaning motion prevents entrance of drainage into nasolacrimal duct.
7. Place curved emesis basin just below client's cheek on side of affected eye.	Basin collects irrigating solution.
8. Fill irrigating syringe or eye dropper. Gently retract lower and upper eyelids (conjunctival sacs) by applying pressure to lower bony orbit and bony prominence beneath eyebrow. Do not apply pressure over eye.	Retraction minimizes blinking and exposes upper and lower conjunctival membranes for irrigation. Pressure on internal eye structures could cause permanent injury.
9. Hold irrigating syringe or dropper approximately 2.5 cm (1 inch) above inner canthus.	If dropper or syringe touches eye, there is risk of injury. Dropper or syringe becomes contaminated.

Steps	Rationale
10. Ask client to look up. Gently irrigate by directing solution into lower conjunctival sac toward outer canthus. Use only enough force to remove secretions gently.	Flushing of conjunctival sac prevents exposure of sensitive cornea to solution. Fluid flows away from nasolacrimal duct, minimizing absorption of contaminated solution.
11. Allow client to close his eye periodically, particularly if burning or excess blinking occurs. Encourage his cooperation.	Lid closure moves secretions from upper to lower conjunctival sac. Also promotes client's ability to relax during procedure.
12. Continue irrigation until all solution is used or secretions have been cleaned. (Remember: a 15-min irrigation is needed to flush chemicals.)	Serves to clean exudate, relieve inflammation, or flush caustic solution.
13. Dry eyelids and facial area with sterile cotton ball. Client may resume normal position.	Removes excess solution and provides for client's comfort.
14. Remove equipment and wash hands.	Reduces transfer of microorganisms.
15. Record in nurse's notes client's response to irrigation (burning, itching, pain) as well as volume and type of solution used, character of drainage, and appearance of conjunctiva.	Timely recording provides accurate documentation of client's response to procedure.

Nurse Alert

Be sure that a client's contact lenses are removed before beginning any irrigation. When caustic chemicals enter the eye, it is necessary to flush the eye continuously for at least 15 minutes. Continuous flushing prevents burning of the sensitive cornea. Do not apply pressure directly on the eye during irrigation. This could injure the eye.

Client Teaching

Clients can be taught to administer eye irrigations at home. However, they may need to use an eye cup, which should be practiced before it is attempted alone.

Pediatric Considerations

Young children are at risk of getting objects in their eyes accidentally during the normal course of play. The parent should act quickly, since a child's natural response is to begin rubbing his eye. It may be necessary to restrain a young child so the eye can be properly and thoroughly irrigated. The easiest technique is to have the child stand over a sink as the parent flushes the eye with tap water.

Geriatric Considerations

An elderly client may have reduced coordination of the hand or fingers and require assistance from an available family member or friend in administering the irrigation. If a client lives alone, he should try to perform the irrigation himself. Any delay could result in burns to the cornea.

Applying an Abdominal Binder (Straight and Scultetus)

Abdominal binders support large abdominal incisions, which are vulnerable to tension or stress as the client moves or coughs. An abdominal binder is a rectangular piece of cotton or elasticized material that has either many tails attached to the two longer sides (as with the scultetus type) or long extensions on each side to surround the abdomen. A properly applied binder provides support and comfort so the client can resume normal activities early.

Potential Nursing Diagnoses

Clients who require an abdominal binder may have one or more of the following nursing diagnoses:

Alteration in comfort related to incisional pain
Impaired skin integrity related to open wound
Impaired physical mobility related to incisional pain
Ineffective breathing patterns related to incisional pain

Equipment

Abdominal binder of size sufficient to surround client's abdomen
Safety pins (optional)

Steps	Rationale
1. Wash hands.	Reduces transmission of microorganisms
2. Explain to client that binder serves to support abdominal incision and provides comfort.	Reduces client's anxiety.
3. Instruct client to roll onto one side while supporting abdominal incision and dressing firmly with hands.	Reduces pain.
4. Place binder (fan folded) under client in same manner as when applying sheet for an occupied bed (Skill 5-22).	Allows client to roll over binder to ease positioning and centering.
5. Have client roll to opposite side. Unfold binder beneath him.	
6. Position client supine over center of binder. Bottom edge of binder should be just above symphysis pubis, and top edge below costal margins.	Ensures that adequate pressure will be applied over wound. Also prevents interference with chest expansion.
7. Close the binder:	Firm even application provides optimal wound support and comfort.

Straight
▪ Pull left end of binder toward center of client's abdomen. While keeping tension on left end, pull right end over left. Secure by smoothing Velcro edges together.

Steps	Rationale

Scultetus
- With your left hand, bring bottom tail at client's left side over toward center of abdomen. Keeping tension on tail, overlap it with bottom right tail. Repeat with each successive pair of tails, moving toward top of binder. Double the ends of tails back on themselves to prevent bulging or pressure areas. Be sure that each pair of tails overlaps pair below. Secure top pair with safety pin for each end. (Fig. 158)

8. Assess client's ability to deep breathe and cough. Readjust as necessary

   Binder should not impair chest expansion or exert increased pressure over abdomen.

9. Wash hands.

   Reduces transmission of microorganisms.

10. Record in nurse's notes application and client's tolerance.

    Prompt documentation improves accuracy of record.

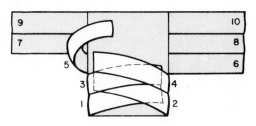

Fig. 158

Nurse Alert

An abdominal binder should apply support to the abdominal structures but should never be so tight as to cause pain or impede deep breathing or coughing.

Client Teaching

Explanation of the procedure promotes client cooperation. In addition, teaching the client about why the binder is necessary can improve his mobility and his deep breathing and coughing.

Geriatric Considerations

An elderly person normally has, as a result of the aging process, reduced chest expansion and a diminished vital capacity. A binder should not restrict his ability to ventilate fully.

Applying an Elastic Roller Bandage

An elastic roller (Ace) bandage is used to apply compression to a knee or ankle (or an elbow or wrist), following strains or sprains. When applied smoothly, it provides excellent support so the affected body part can be used without further risk of injury. The Ace bandage is also used to wrap amputated extremities during the healing phase to prevent edema.

Potential Nursing Diagnoses

Clients requiring an Ace bandage may have one or more of the following nursing diagnoses:

Impaired physical mobility related to muscle sprain
Impaired physical mobility related to amputated extremity
Potential or actual impairment of skin integrity related to trauma
Alteration in comfort related to muscle strain

Equipment

Elastic (Ace) bandage
Rolled gauze (optional)
Tape or metal stays

Steps	Rationale
1. Wash hands.	Reduces transmission of microorganisms.
2. Stand in front of body part to be bandaged.	Improves access and facilitates handling bandage.

Steps	Rationale
3. Hold free end of bandage in your nondominant hand and place its outer surface against client's skin. Hold body of bandage in your dominant hand. (Fig. 159)	Holding body of bandage with outer surface against client's skin improves ease of unrolling remainder of bandage.
4. With firm even tension, wrap bandage around distal portion of body part, anchoring free end of bandage. (Fig. 160)	Application from distal end toward trunk promotes venous return. Anchoring bandage end prevents slippage.
5. Pass body of bandage from hand to hand while making even spiral turns up body part. (Each turn overlaps previous turn by half or two thirds width of bandage.)	Gradual and even unwinding applies equal pressure to body part.
6. Once full roll of bandage is applied, secure terminal end with tape or metal stays.	Prevents slippage. Tape and stays do not place pressure against client's skin.
7. Assess circulation and sensation of distal body part.	Too firm an application can impair blood flow.

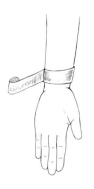

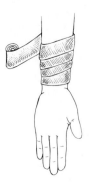

Fig. 159   Fig. 160

Steps	Rationale
8. Record in nurse's notes extremity or body part bandaged and adequacy of circulation in distal body part.	Documents circulation to distal extremity following application of bandage.

Nurse Alert

Continual assessment of tissues distal to the dressing for signs of circulatory impairment is necessary to provide a means of comparing changes in circulation after bandage application. Circulatory impairment is identified by coolness, pallor or cyanosis (bluish discoloration), diminished or absent pulses, swelling, numbness, and tingling (paresthesia).

Client Teaching

Clients are frequently discharged with elastic bandages. However, they should be taught how to apply the bandage and the signs of circulatory impairment. In addition, they should be given an opportunity to demonstrate their skill at wrapping the affected body part.

Geriatric Considerations

Older adults are often at risk of peripheral circulatory impairment as well as skin breakdown due to pressure. When an elastic bandage is essential, the nurse must first document the status of the client's pulses and the integrity of the skin. Once the bandage is applied, more frequent assessments will be needed.

Applying a Hot Moist Compress to an Open Wound

A hot moist compress is effective for improving circulation, relieving edema, and promoting the consolidation and drainage of pus. Because the compress is applied to an open wound, it must be sterile.

Potential Nursing Diagnoses

Clients who require a hot moist compress may have one or more of the following nursing diagnoses:

Potential for injury related to an open wound

Impaired mobility related to painful incision

Alteration in comfort related to incisional wound

Equipment

Prescribed solution warmed to proper temperature (approximately 43°-46° C [110°-115° F])

Sterile gauze dressings

Sterile container for solution

Commercially prepared compresses (optional)

Sterile gloves

Petrolatum jelly

Sterile cotton swabs

Waterproof pad

Tape or ties

Dry bath towel

Water-flow or heating pad (optional)
Disposable gloves
Bath thermometer

Steps	Rationale
1. Explain procedure to client, including sensations to be felt (e.g., feeling of warmth and wetness). Explain precautions to prevent burning.	Improves client cooperation and lessens anxiety
2. Assist client to comfortable position in proper body alignment.	Compress will remain in place for several minutes. Limited mobility in uncomfortable position can cause muscular stress.
3. Place waterproof pad under area to be treated.	Prevents soiling of bed linen.
4. Expose body part to be covered with compress. Drape rest of body with bath blanket.	Prevents unnecessary cooling and exposure of body part.
5. Wash hands.	Reduces transmission of infection.
6. Assemble equipment. Pour warmed solution in sterile container. (If using a portable heating source, keep solution warm. Commercially prepared compresses may remain under infrared lamp until just before use.) Open sterile packages and drop gauze into container to become immersed in solution. Turn electrical heating pad to correct temperature.	Compresses must retain warmth for therapeutic benefit.

Steps	Rationale
7. Don disposable gloves. Remove any dressings covering wound. Dispose of gloves and dressings in proper receptacle.	Proper disposal prevents spread of microorganisms.
8. Assess condition of wound and surrounding skin.	Provides baseline for determining skin changes after compress application.
9. Don sterile gloves.	Sterile touching sterile remains sterile.
10. Apply petrolatum jelly with a cotton swab to skin surrounding wound. Do not place jelly on areas of broken skin.	Protects skin from possible burns and maceration (softening).
11. Pick up one layer of immersed gauze and wring out any excess water.	Excess moisture macerates skin and increases risk of burns and infection.
12. Apply gauze lightly to open wound. Watch client's response and ask if he feels discomfort. In a few seconds, lift edge of gauze to assess skin for redness.	Skin is most sensitive to sudden change in temperature. Redness indicates a burn.
13. If client tolerates hot compress, pack gauze snugly against wound. Be sure that all wound surfaces are covered.	Packing of compress prevents rapid cooling from underlying air currents.
14. Wrap moist compress with dry bath towel. If necessary, pin or tie in place.	Insulates compress to prevent heat loss.
15. Change the hot compress every 5 minutes.	Prevents cooling, thus maintaining therapeutic benefit of compress.

Steps	Rationale
16. (Optional) Apply water-flow or waterproof heating pad over towel. Keep it in place for desired duration of application (usually 20-30 min).	Provides constant temperature to compress.
17. Ask client periodically if there is any discomfort or burning sensation.	Continued exposure to heat can cause burning of skin.
18. Remove pad, towel, and compress. Assess wound and condition of surrounding skin.	Continued exposure to moisture will macerate skin.
19. Replace sterile dressing.	Prevents entrance of microorganisms into wound site.
20. Dispose of equipment and wash hands.	
21. Record in nurse's notes type of application, solution, temperature of solution, duration of application, and condition of skin before and after procedure.	Accurate documentation protects you legally.

Nurse Alert

The nurse must use caution to avoid burning the client's skin. Because moisture conducts heat, the temperature setting on any device applied to a moist compress need not be as high as if the device is used for a dry application.

Client Teaching

Clients may frequently use compresses or heating devices in the house. Instruct them on ways to avoid burns: always time applications carefully to avoid overexposure; do not adjust the temperature of a heating pad to a high setting; do not lie directly on a heating device but instead apply it to the skin.

Pediatric Considerations

When applying a hot moist compress to a child, determine the need to restrain him so he does not contaminate the wound. If possible, you may use this time to cuddle and read to the child so as not to dislodge the compress.

Geriatric Considerations

Elderly persons frequently suffer a loss of or reduction in temperature sensation due to aging or chronic disease. Therefore, watch the client's skin condition carefully during heat application.

Assisting a Client With IPPB Therapy

Intermittent positive pressure breathing (IPPB) therapy is selected to optimize airway patency and promote deep breathing. In addition it can be used to deliver medications to the airways.

Potential Nursing Diagnoses

Clients who require IPPB therapy may have one or more of the following nursing diagnoses:

Ineffective airway clearance related to airway secretions

Impaired gas exchange related to decreased chest wall movements

Ineffective airway clearance related to diminished cough

Equipment

IPPB machine
Oxygen tubing
Nebulizer
Oxygen source

Steps	Rationale
1. Explain procedure to client and have him practice using mouthpiece before procedure.	Reduces procedure-related anxiety. Practice assists client in becoming accustomed to airtight seal that he must create with his lips for IPPB machine to work correctly.
2. Place client in high Fowler position.	Promotes optimal lung expansion.

Steps	Rationale
3. Encourage him to relax during inspiratory cycle.	Promotes optimal lung expansion.
4. Encourage him to exhale normally.	Exhalation is usually twice as long as inspiration. IPPB machine is preset to click on with client's normal beginning inspiratory maneuvers.
5. If client is breathing through his nose and is not able to breathe entirely through his mouth, a nose clip may be needed.	Nose clips produce an airtight seal needed for IPPB system to function effectively. NOTE: Some clients may experience sensation of claustrophopia with nose clip, and their anxiety is increased.
6. Observe client's chest wall movements. If they are asymmetrical or if chest pain occurs, stop procedure and assess client's respiratory system.	Early identification of barotrauma may be indicated by asymmetrical chest wall movement or chest pain.
7. Observe any sputum production after treatment.	Discolored sputum indicates pulmonary infection. If discolored sputum is a new finding, it should be reported.
8. Change oxygen tubes and nebulizer every 24 hours.	Risk of nosocomial (hospital acquired) infection is reduced when oxygen tubes and nebulizer are changed every 24 hours.
9. Record in nurse's notes time and duration of treatment, as well as client's response.	Documents that client did receive therapy.

Nurse Alert

If barotrauma is suspected, notify the physician and do a complete respiratory and vital signs assessment on the client.

Client Teaching

Clients must be instructed to breathe with the cycle of the IPPB machine. The synchronization of respirations will be easier if the client has been instructed in relaxation techniques prior to IPPB therapy. These techniques include diaphragmatic breathing and progressive muscle relaxation.

Pediatric Considerations

IPPB therapy is not used frequently with children. For IPPB therapy to be effective there must be full cooperation by the client. Children are usually unable to cooperate fully with IPPB therapy.

Geriatric Considerations

IPPB therapy should not be used with confused or fearful clients because of their inability to fully cooperate.

Postural Drainage

Postural drainage is the gravitational clearance of airway secretions from specific bronchial segments. It is achieved by assuming one or more of 10 different body positions. Each position drains a specific section of the tracheobronchial tree—the upper, middle, or lower lung field—into the trachea. Coughing or suctioning can then remove secretions from the trachea. The figures and list on the next pages show the bronchial area and the corresponding body posture for its drainage.

Potential Nursing Diagnoses

Clients requiring postural drainage may have one or more of the following nursing diagnoses:

Ineffective airway clearance related to impaired cough

Ineffective breathing patterns related to decreased lung expansion

Impaired gas exchange related to retained airway secretions

Equipment

Pillows—two to three extra

Slant or tilt board (if drainage to be performed in home)

Facial tissues

Glass of water

Clear jar

Positions for Postural Drainage

Left and Right Upper Lobe Anterior Apical Bronchi

Have client sit in chair, leaning back against pillow.
(Figs. 161, 162)

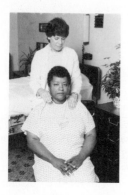

Fig. 161

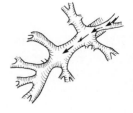

Fig. 162

Left and Right Upper Lobe Posterior Apical Bronchi

Have client sit in chair, leaning forward on pillow or table.
(Figs. 163, 164)

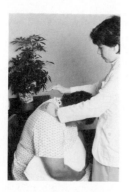

Fig. 163

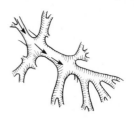

Fig. 164

Right and Left Anterior Upper Lobe Bronchi

Have client lie flat on back with small pillow under knees. (Figs. 165, 166)

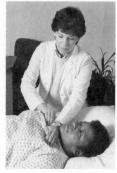

Fig. 165

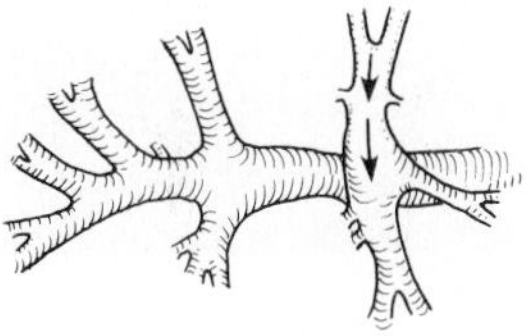

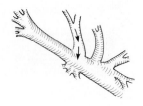

Fig. 166

Left Upper Lobe Lingual Bronchus

Have client lie on right side with arm over head in Trendelenburg position, with foot of bed raised 30 cm (12 inches). Place pillow behind back, and roll client one fourth turn onto pillow. (Figs. 167, 168)

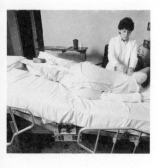

Fig. 167

Fig. 168

Right Middle Lobe Bronchus

Have client lie on left side and raise foot of bed 30 cm (12 inches). Place pillow behind back and roll client one fourth turn onto pillow.
(Figs. 169, 170)

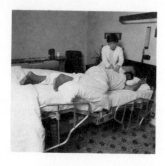

Fig. 169

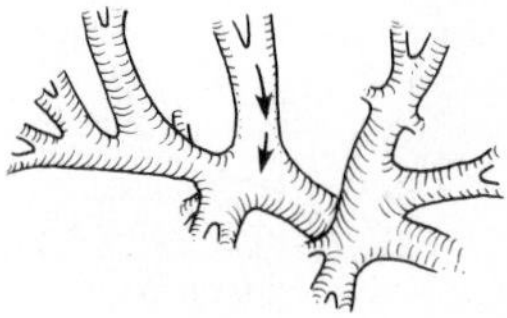

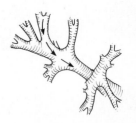

Fig. 170

Left and Right Anterior Lower Lobe Bronchi

Have client lie on back in Trendelenburg position, with foot of bed elevated 45-50 cm (18-20 inches). Have knees bent on pillow.
(Figs. 171, 172)

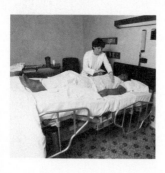

Fig. 171

Fig. 172

Right Lower Lobe Lateral Bronchus

Have client lie on left side in Trendelenburg position with foot
of bed raised 45-50 cm (18-20 inches).
(Figs. 173, 174)

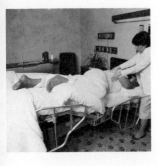

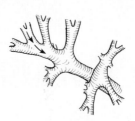

Fig. 173   Fig. 174

Left Lower Lobe Lateral Bronchus

Have client lie on right side in Trendelenburg position with foot
of bed raised 45-50 cm (18-20 inches).
(Figs. 175, 176)

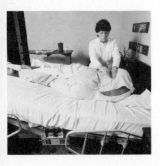

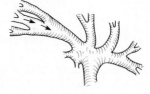

Fig. 175   Fig. 176

Right and Left Lower Lobe Superior Bronchi

Have client lie flat on stomach with pillow under stomach. (Figs. 177, 178)

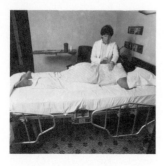

Fig. 177   Fig. 178

Left and Right Posterior Basal Bronchi

Have client lie on stomach in Trendelenburg position with foot of bed elevated 45-50 cm (18-20 inches). (Figs. 179, 180)

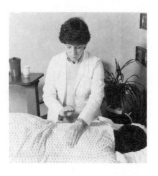

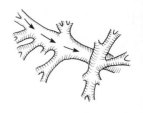

Fig. 179   Fig. 180

Steps	Rationale
1. Wash hands.	Reduces transmission of microorganisms.
2. Select congested areas to be drained based on assessment of all lung fields, clinical data, and chest x-ray views.	To be effective, treatment must be individualized to treat specific areas involved.

Steps	Rationale
3. Place client in position to drain congested areas. (First area selected may vary from client to client.) Help client assume position as needed. Teach client correct posture and arm and leg positioning. Place pillows for support and comfort.	Specific positions are selected to drain each area involved.
4. Have client maintain posture for 10-15 minutes.	In adults, draining each area takes time. In children, 3-5 minutes is sufficient.
5. During 10-15 minutes of drainage in this posture, perform chest percussion, vibration, and/or rib shaking over area being drained.	Provides mechanical forces that aid in mobilization of airway secretions.
6. After drainage in first posture, have client sit up and cough. Save expectorated secretions in clear container. If client cannot cough, suctioning should be performed.	Any secretions mobilized into central airways should be removed by cough and/or suctioning before client is placed in next drainage position. Coughing is most effective when client is sitting up and leaning forward.
7. Have client rest briefly if necessary.	Short rest periods between postures can prevent fatigue and help client to better tolerate therapy.
8. Have client take sips of water.	Keeping mouth moist aids in expectoration of secretions.
9. Repeat Steps 3 to 8 until all congested areas selected have been drained. Each treatment should not exceed 30-60 minutes.	Postural drainage is used only to drain areas involved and is based on individual assessment.

Steps	Rationale
10. Repeat chest assessment of all lung fields.	Allows you to assess need for further drainage or changes in drainage program.
11. Wash your hands.	Reduces transmission of microorganisms.

Nurse Alert

Bronchospasm can be induced in some clients receiving postural drainage. It is caused by mobilization of secretions into the large central airways, which increases the work of breathing. To counteract the risk of bronchospasm, the nurse may ask the physician to start the client on bronchodilator therapy 20 minutes before postural drainage.

Client Teaching

The client and family should be taught how to assume postures at home. Some postures may need to be modified to meet individual needs. For example, the side-lying Trendelenburg position to drain the lateral lower lobes may have to be done with the client lying flat on his side or in a side-lying semi-Fowler position if he is very short of breath (dyspneic).

Pediatric Considerations

It is unrealistic to expect a child to cooperate fully in assuming all positions used for postural drainage. The nurse should set four to six positions as priority. More than six will frequently exceed the child's limit of tolerance.

Geriatric Considerations

Clients on antihypertensive medication may not be able to tolerate the postural changes required. The nurse must then modify the procedure to meet the client's tolerance and still clear his airways.

Oropharyngeal and Nasopharyngeal Suctioning

Oropharyngeal or nasopharyngeal suctioning is used when the client is able to cough effectively but is unable to clear secretions by expectorating or swallowing. It is frequently used after the client has coughed. Oropharyngeal and nasopharyngeal suction may also be appropriate in less responsive or comatose clients who require removal of oral secretions.

Potential Nursing Diagnoses

Clients requiring oropharyngeal or nasopharyngeal suctioning may have one or more of the following nursing diagnoses:

Ineffective airway clearance related to impaired cough reflex

Ineffective airway clearance related to immobility

Potential for injury related to pulmonary aspiration

Equipment

Portable or wall suction unit with connecting tubing and Y connector if needed

Sterile catheter (12 or 16 French)

Sterile water or normal saline

Sterile gloves

Drape or towel to protect linen and client's bedclothes

Steps	Rationale
1. Prepare equipment at bedside.	Allows smooth performance of procedure without interruption.
2. Wash hands.	Reduces transmission of microorganisms.
3. Explain to client how procedure will help clear airway and relieve some of his breathing problems. Explain that coughing, sneezing, or gagging is normal.	
4. Properly position client: ▪ If conscious with a functional gag reflex—Place him in semi-Fowler position with head turned to one side for oral suctioning. Place him in semi-Fowler position with neck hyperextended for nasal suctioning.	Gag reflex helps prevent aspiration of gastrointestinal contents. Positioning head to one side or hyperextending neck promotes smooth insertion of catheter into oropharynx or nasopharynx respectively.
▪ If unconscious—Place him in lateral position facing you for oral or nasal suctioning.	Prevents client's tongue from obstructing airway, promotes drainage of pulmonary secretions, and prevents aspiration of gastrointestinal contents.
5. Place towel on pillow or under client's chin.	Soiling of bed linen or bed clothes from secretions is prevented. Towel can be discarded, reducing spread of bacteria.
6. Select proper suction pressure and the type of suction unit. For wall suction units this is 120-150 mm Hg in adults,	Assures safe negative pressure according to client's age. Excessive negative pressure can precipitate. injury to mucosa.

Steps	Rationale
100-120 mm Hg in children, or 60-100 mm Hg in infants.	
7. Pour sterile water or saline into sterile container.	Needed to lubricate catheter to decrease friction and promote smooth passage.
8. Put sterile glove on your dominant hand.	Maintains asepsis as catheter is passed into client's mouth or nose.
9. Using your gloved hand, attach catheter to suction machine.	Sterility is maintained
10. Approximate the distance between client's earlobe and tip of nose and place thumb and forefinger of your gloved hand at that point.	This distance ensures that suction catheter will remain in pharyngeal region. Insertion of catheter past this point places catheter in trachea.
11. Moisten catheter tip with sterile solution. Apply suction with tip in solution.	Moistening catheter tip reduces friction and eases insertion. Applying suction while catheter is in sterile solution ensures that suction equipment is functioning before catheter is inserted.
12. Suction	
▪ Oropharyngeal—Gently insert catheter into one side of client's mouth and guide it to oropharynx. Do not apply suction during insertion.	Stimulation of gag reflex is reduced.
▪ Nasopharyngeal—Gently insert catheter into one naris. Guide it medially along floor of nasal cavity. Do not force catheter. If one	Catheter avoids nasal turbinates and enters more easily into nasopharynx. Risk of trauma to oral and nasal mucosa during catheter insertion is reduced.

Steps	Rationale
naris is not patent, try other. Do not apply suction during insertion.	
13. Occlude suction port with your thumb. Gently rotate catheter as you withdraw it. Entire procedure should not take longer than 15 seconds.	Occlusion of suction port activates suction pressure. Suctioning is intermittently done as catheter is withdrawn. Rotation removes secretions from all surfaces of airway and prevents trauma from suction pressure on one area of airway. NOTE: Suctioning also removes air. Client's oxygen supply can be severely reduced if procedure lasts longer than 15 seconds.
14. Flush catheter with sterile solution by placing it in solution and applying suction.	Removes secretions from catheter and lubricates it for next suctioning.
15. If client is not in respiratory distress, allow him to rest for 20-30 seconds before reinserting catheter.	Allows client opportunity to increase his oxygen intake.
16. If client is able, ask him to deep breathe and cough between suctions.	Promotes mobilization of secretions to upper airway, where they can be removed with catheter. If client is able to cough productively, further suctioning may not be needed so long as his airways are clear to auscultation.
17. If resuctioning is needed, repeat Steps 11 through 13.	
18. Suction secretions in mouth or under tongue after suctioning oropharynx or nasopharynx.	Sterile asepsis is maintained. Mouth should be suctioned only after sterile areas have been thoroughly suctioned.

Steps	Rationale
19. Discard catheter by wrapping it around your gloved hand and pulling glove off around catheter.	Spread of bacteria from suction catheter is reduced.
20. Prepare equipment for next suctioning.	Ready access to suction equipment is provided, especially if the client is experiencing respiratory distress.
21. Record in nurse's notes amount, consistency, color, and odor of secretions as well as client's response to procedure.	Documents that procedure was completed.

Nurse Alert

If the client is unable to cough or has an artificial airway, orotracheal or nasotracheal suctioning is necessary.

Client Teaching

Clients who have undergone head and neck surgery (such as laryngectomy or neck dissection) often learn to self-administer oral suctioning while in the hospital. This can give them a sense of independence.

Pediatric Considerations

Children require smaller-diameter suction catheters. The newborn to 18-month-old child requires a 6 to 8 French, the 18-to-24-month old an 8 to 10 French, and the older child a 10 to 14 French.

Geriatric Considerations

Elderly clients with underlying cardiac or pulmonary disease may be able to tolerate only a 10-second period of suctioning. These clients are at greater risk of hypoxia-induced cardiac arrhythmias.

Applying a Nasal Cannula

A nasal cannula is a simple device that can be inserted into the nares for delivery of oxygen and that allows the client to breathe through his mouth or nose. It is available for all age groups and is adequate for both short- and long-term use in the hospital or at home.

Potential Nursing Diagnoses

Clients requiring oxygen delivery by way of a nasal cannula may have one or more of the following nursing diagnoses:

Impaired gas exchange related to decreased lung expansion
Impaired gas exchange related to inadequate oxygen intake
Impaired gas exchange related to airway secretions

Equipment

Nasal cannula
Oxygen tubing
Humidifier
Oxygen source with flowmeter
"No smoking" signs

Steps	Rationale
1. Wash hands	Reduces transmission of microorganisms.
2. Attach cannula to oxygen tubing.	Establishes connection with oxygen source. Oxygen tubing has extension length so client has some mobility.

447

Steps	Rationale
3. Adjust oxygen flow to prescribed rate, usually between 1 and 6 L/min. Observe that water in humidifier is bubbling.	Administers oxygen at prescribed rate. Oxygen flow rates greater than 6 L/min do not increase oxygen concentration but do irritate nasal mucosa, causing swallowing of gas and abdominal distention.
4. Place prongs of cannula in client's nose and adjust band to client's comfort. (Fig. 181)	Reduces chance that client will remove cannula because of discomfort.
5. Check cannula every 8 hours.	Patency of cannula and oxygen flow are ensured.
6. Keep humidification jar filled at all times.	Inhalation of dehumidified oxygen is prevented.
7. Assess client's nares, external nose, and ears for mucosal and/or skin breakdown every 6-8 hours.	Prolonged use of nasal oxygen can increase risk of mucosal breakdown in nares. Tape can irritate bridge of nose. Elastic band can excoriate ears.
8. Check oxygen flow rate and physician's orders every 8 hours.	Delivery of prescribed oxygen flow rate is ensured.

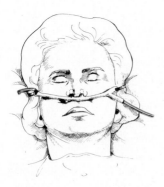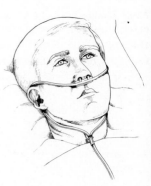

Fig. 181

Steps	Rationale
9. Record in client's record time that therapy was initiated, oxygen flow rate, route of administration, and client's response.	Documents that procedure was performed.

Nurse Alert

In clients with underlying obstructive lung disease the flow rate of oxygen should not exceed 2 L/min. Higher rates can depress the stimulus to breathe.

Client Teaching

Clients may be placed on home oxygen via nasal cannula. They and their families must then be taught the hazards of oxygen therapy, the rationale for it, the correct flow rate, and the proper use and cleaning of oxygen equipment.

Pediatric Considerations

In general, oxygen is delivered via an oxygen tent to a child.

Geriatric Considerations

Frail elderly clients are at increased risk of skin breakdown resulting from the placement of an oxygen cannula. The sites for skin breakdown include the nares and ears. Skin breakdown can be minimized by frequent assessment of and care to these areas.

Inserting a Nasal Catheter

A nasal catheter is a soft tube that can be inserted into the nose for delivery of oxygen. Although it is used less frequently than a cannula or oxygen mask, it is not obsolete. Nasal catheters can cause discomfort, become lodged in the nasal cavity, and lead to excessive oropharyngeal drying.

Potential Nursing Diagnoses

Clients requiring oxygen delivery by way of a nasal cannula may have one or more of the following nursing diagnoses:

Impaired gas exchange related to inadequate oxygen intake

Impaired gas exchange related to airway secretions

Impaired gas exchange related to decreased level of consciousness

Equipment

Appropriate size of nasal catheter: small diameter (8 or 10 gauge French) for children; larger diameter (10 or 14 gauge French) for adults

Oxygen tubing

Humidifier

Oxygen source with flowmeter

Lubricating jelly (must be water soluble)

Nonallergenic tape

Flashlight or penlight

Tongue depressor

"No smoking" signs

Steps	Rationale
1. Wash hands.	Reduces transmission of microorganisms.
2. Prepare equipment at bedside.	Ensures completion of procedure without interruption.
3. Verify physician's order for oxygen flow rate, method of delivery, and nasal catheter.	Ensures that right amount of oxygen is administered via right route to right client.
4. Explain procedure to client, emphasizing why neither client nor visitors can smoke in the presence of oxygen.	Reduces client's anxiety and promotes safety by preventing fires.
5. Place "no smoking" signs on client's wall at head of bed and outside door.	Notifies all personnel and visitors that oxygen is in use. Maintains client safety.
6. Assist client to semi-Fowler or high Fowler position.	Work of breathing is decreased by allowing for maximal lung expansion.
7. Attach catheter to oxygen tubing, and oxygen tubing to humidifier.	Oxygen must be humidified to prevent consolidation of pulmonary secretions.

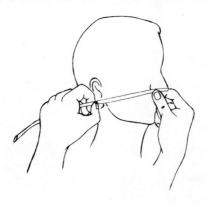

Fig. 182

Steps	Rationale
8. Measure proper length of tubing to be inserted: distance from client's nose to earlobe. Mark point with piece of tape. (Fig. 182)	Approximates distance to oropharynx.
9. Lubricate tip of catheter with water-soluble jelly.	Lipid-base lubrication should never be used, since if aspirated it could cause severe lung irritation and pneumonia.
10. Set flow rate at 2-3 L/min before inserting catheter.	Prevents plugging of catheter by secretions during insertion.
11. Gently place catheter in one nostril. Guide it medially along floor of nasal cavity. Stop at premarked point. (Fig. 183)	Promotes smooth passage past nasal turbinates and into oropharynx.
12. Inspect oral cavity using tongue depressor and flashlight. Tip of catheter should be visible on either side of uvula. (Fig. 184)	Verifies that catheter is in oropharynx.
13. Withdraw catheter tip so it is no longer visible.	Reduces amount of air swallowed.

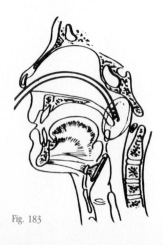

Fig. 183

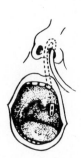

Fig. 184

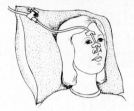

Fig. 185

Steps	Rationale
14. Secure catheter to client's nose.	Prevents displacement.
15. Readjust flow rate to prescribed setting.	Ensures that prescribed amount of oxygen is delivered.
16. Secure tubing to client's pillow, allowing for slack. (Fig. 185)	Client must be able to move without displacing catheter.
17. Assess client's respiratory status after procedure.	Provides data about how client has tolerated procedure and therapy.
18. Record in nurse's notes when procedure was begun, oxygen flow rate, route of administration, and client's response.	Documents that procedure was performed.

Nurse Alert

The flow rate of oxygen should not exceed 2 to 3 L/min in clients with underlying obstructive lung disease. Higher levels of oxygen can depress the stimulus to breathe. Furthermore, because securing the catheter can cause pressure on the naris, the catheter must be changed every 8 hours and inserted into the other naris. As a result, nasal catheters are not as frequently used as they once were.

Cardiopulmonary

Resuscitation

(Two Nurses)

The purpose of cardiopulmonary resuscitation (CPR) is to restore an airway, breathing, and circulation to a client who has sustained catastrophic disruption of these functions.

Cardiopulmonary arrest is characterized by an absence of pulse and respirations and by dilated pupils. CPR is a basic emergency procedure for life support, consisting of artificial respiration and manual external cardiac massage.

Potential Nursing Diagnoses

Clients requiring CPR can have one or more of the following nursing diagnoses:

Decreased cardiac output related to absence or irregularity of heartbeat

Impaired gas exchange related to inadequate respirations

Impaired tissue perfusion

Equipment

Oral airway if immediately available

Automatic manual breathing unit (AMBU) bag if immediately available

Steps	Rationale
1. Determine if pulse and respirations are absent.	Indicates absence of spontaneous cardiopulmonary function.
2. If immediately available, obtain AMBU bag with face mask and oxygen connecting tube.	Produces consistent lung volumes with each artificial respiration.
3. Place client on a hard surface, such as floor, or use a backboard.	External compression of heart is facilitated. Heart is compressed between sternum and hard surface.
4. Maintain open airway by hyperextending neck. Place one hand behind victim's neck and other on forehead. (Fig. 186) ■ Lift neck and apply pressure on forehead. Do not hyperextend neck if spinal cord injury is suspected. Use jaw thrust maneuver. ■ If victim is a child, tilt head backward only slightly. (Fig. 187)	Relieves airway obstruction from tongue, providing clear passage for ventilation.
5. Begin artificial respiration: ■ For mouth-to-mouth resuscitation of adult, pinch victim's nose and	Airtight seal is formed and air does not escape from nose.

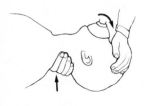

Fig. 186

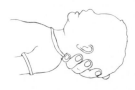

Fig. 187

Steps	Rationale
occlude his mouth with yours. For child, place your mouth over child's nose and mouth. (Fig. 188)	
■ For AMBU bag resuscitation, use proper-size face mask and apply it over victim's mouth and nose. (Fig. 189)	Airtight seal is formed as bag is compressed and oxygen enters victim.
6. Administer artificial respiration:	
■ For mouth-to-mouth resuscitation of adult, blow four quick breaths into victim's mouth. Each breath should have increasing volume and strength. Allow victim to exhale passively. Then administer one breath every 5 seconds.	Promotes hyperoxygenation and assists in maintaining blood oxygen levels.
■ For mouth-to-mouth resuscitation of child, administer short puffs from cheeks once every 3 seconds.	Prevents overinflation of child's lungs with adult volumes.

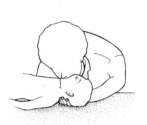

Fig. 188

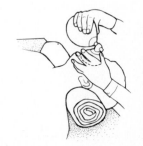

Fig. 189

Steps	Rationale
▪ For artificial respiration with AMBU bag in adult, compress bag fully for four breaths. Repeat every 5 seconds.	Promotes hyperoxygenation and assists in maintaining blood oxygen levels.
▪ For AMBU bag resuscitation in child, perform quick, small compressions of bag every 3 seconds.	Prevents overinflation of child's lungs.
7. Observe for rise and fall of chest wall with each respiration. If lungs do not inflate, reposition head and neck and check for visible airway obstruction, such as vomitus.	Ensures that artificial respirations are entering the lungs.
8. Suction any secretions from airway. If suction is unavailable, turn victim's head to one side.	Prevents airway obstruction. Turning victim's head to one side allows gravity to drain secretions.
9. Assess presence of carotid pulse. Absence of or questionable pulse indicates need for external cardiac compression.	Presence and quality of pulse are ensured.
10. Begin external cardiac compression: *Adult* ▪ Locate xiphoid process (below sternum). Place heel of one hand 4-5 cm (1½-2 inches) above xiphoid process. Place heel of other hand over first hand.	Compressions directly over xiphoid process can lacerate victim's liver.

Steps	Rationale
▪ Keep hands parallel and fingers away from victim's chest. Fingers may be interlocked. Keep elbows extended.	Compression occurs only on sternum. Pressure necessary for external compression is created by your upper arm muscles.
▪ Compress chest 4-5 cm (2-2½ inches) once every second. Count one, one thousand, two, one thousand, etc.	Sixty compressions a minute should be delivered to ensure adequate cardiac output.
▪ Ventilate lungs after each fifth compression. *Infant and small child*	Promotes adequate ventilation during CPR.
▪ Compress sternum 1-2 cm (½-1 inch) with both thumbs while supporting back, or use fingertips of index and middle fingers of one hand. (Figs. 190, 191)	Prevents damage to external structures from excessive pressure.
▪ Deliver 80-100 compressions every minute.	Simulates more rapid heart rate of infants and children.
▪ Ventilate lungs every 3 seconds.	Promotes adequate ventilation during CPR.
11. Palpate for carotid pulse with each external chest compression.	Validates that adequate stroke volume is achieved with each compression.

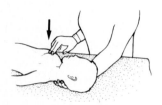

Fig. 190

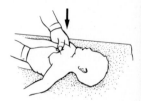

Fig. 191

Steps	Rationale
12. If carotid pulse is not palpable, compressions are not strong enough. Continue CPR until relieved or until victim regains spontaneous pulse and respirations.	Artificial cardiopulmonary function is maintained.

Nurse Alert

If CPR must be interrupted, the interruption should not last longer than 5 to 30 seconds. CPR is interrupted when changing personnel, during defibrillation, or when transporting the victim. The nurse should remind rescue team members of the number of seconds elapsing.

FLUIDS

Measuring and Recording Intake and Output

Measuring and recording all liquid intake and output during a 24-hour period provides a reliable measure of a client's fluid balance. Intake includes all liquids ingested orally and/or administered by feeding tube or parenterally. Liquid output includes urine, diarrhea, vomitus, gastric suction, and drainage from tubes (such as chest tubes or Penrose drains). Any major differences between a client's expected 24-hour intake and output may dictate medical therapy.

Potential Nursing Diagnoses

Clients requiring intake and output measurements may have one or more of the following nursing diagnoses:

Fluid volume excess

Fluid volume deficit

Equipment

Metric cylinder

Bedpan

Urinal

Pencil

Steps	Rationale
1. Explain to client (or family) why intake and output measurements are important.	Ambulatory clients often need to be actively involved. If they have coffee or juice in hospital cafeteria, for example, they can record their own intake.
2. Give client a copy of hospital's metric conversions or a chart adapted to home measurements.·	Provides easy and accurate conversion method for recording intake.
3. Instruct client not to empty urinal, Foley drainage bag, bedpan, or commode but to ask nurse to empty container and record amount.	Maintains accurate record of output.
4. Ask client (or family) to record each episode of urination and whether amount was small, moderate, or large.	Toward end of a postoperative or postpartum period, frequency of voiding is recorded with approximation of amount voided.
5. Compare 24-hour intake with total output.	Determines fluid balance alterations.
6. Record volume of intake and output on flow sheet.	Data used for medical assessment of client's condition.
7. Instruct client or family to contact nursing agency or physician if imbalances occur between intake and output.	Prompt reporting of intake and output imbalances can help prevent severe fluid and electrolyte disturbances.
8. Wash hands after each time urinal or bedpan is handled.	Reduces transmission of microorganisms.

Nurse Alert

The nurse should be alert to changes in the client's liquid intake and output. Average urinary output for a 70 kg (155-pound) adult is 1500 ml, and his intake should be twice that (3000 ml). A guideline for monitoring fluid balance is that intake should be twice output.

Client Teaching

Clients and their families should be taught how to measure and evaluate intake and output. In addition, they should be given guidelines as to when to call the visiting nurse or physician regarding actual or potential fluid imbalances.

Pediatric Considerations

Fluid imbalances, such as dehydration from diarrhea and vomiting, can quickly develop in infants and young children. It is important to accurately assess all output either by a pediatric collection device or by weighing all diapers. An infant's kidneys are functionally immature at birth and thus unable to concentrate or dilute urine.

Geriatric Considerations

Fluid and electrolyte imbalances can also develop quickly in elderly persons, particularly those with cardiac or renal disease. To avoid a serious fluid imbalance, the nurse must continually assess fluid status and monitor intake and output in elderly clients with unstable health status.

Venipuncture

Venipuncture is a technique in which a vein is punctured transcutaneously by a sharp rigid stylet (such as with a butterfly needle, an angiocatheter, a needle attached to a syringe, or a Vacutainer). The general purposes of venipuncture are to collect blood, instill a medication, start an intravenous infusion, or inject a radiopaque substance for x-ray examination of a body part or system. The present skill deals with obtaining a blood specimen. Skill 12-3 discusses venipuncture for the purpose of initiating an intravenous infusion.

Nursing Diagnoses

Clients who undergo venipuncture may have any of the following nursing diagnoses:

Potential for injury related to venipuncture
Alteration in comfort
Potential alteration in skin integrity
Anxiety related to impending venipuncture

Equipment

Specimen tubes
Alcohol and Betadine (povidone-iodine) cleaning swabs
Rubber tourniquet
Towel to place under client's arm
Sterile gauze pads (2 × 2)
Band-Aid or adhesive tape
Syringe method
Sterile needles (20 to 21 gauge for adult; 23 to 25 gauge for child)
Sterile syringe of appropriate size

Vacutainer method
Vacutainer tube with needle holder
Sterile double-ended needles

Steps	Rationale
1. Wash hands.	Reduces transmission of microorganisms.
2. Gather all equipment needed and bring to client.	Maintains organization and avoids having to leave client while you get more equipment.
3. Close bedside curtain or room door.	Provides for client's privacy.
4. Organize equipment on clutter-free surface.	Reduces risk of contamination and accidents.
5. Assist client to supine or semi-Fowler position with his arm extended straight. Place small towel under upper arm.	Stabilizes client's arm and provides easy access to venipuncture site.
6. Open sterile packages using sterile technique.	Prevents contamination of sterile objects.
7. Select distal site in vein to be used. Veins frequently used for blood sampling include those in antecubital fossa and those in lower arm.	If sclerosing or other damage occurs to vein, proximal site in same vein is still usable.
8. If possible, place client's arm in dependent position.	Permits venous dilation, thereby improving visability of vein.
9. Place tourniquet 5-15 cm (2-6 inches) above venipuncture site. Encircle client's arm and pull one end of tourniquet tightly over other, looping one end under other. Do not use a knot.	Allows vein to distend with blood, for better visibility. Permits quick release of tourniquet with one hand.

Steps	Rationale
10. Palpate distal pulse below tourniquet.	Pressure from tourniquet should not impede arterial flow.
11. Select well-dilated vein. It may help to have client make fist. Do not keep tourniquet on longer than 1-2 minutes.	Muscle contraction increases venous distention. Prolonged tourniquet time may cause venous stasis and thereby alter test results.
12. Clean venipuncture site with povidone-iodine (Betadine) solution and follow with alcohol. Move in circular motion out from site approximately 5 cm (2 inches).	Betadine is a topical anti-infective; alcohol, a topical antiseptic. Together these agents reduce skin surface bacteria.
13. Remove needle cover from syringe or Vacutainer and inform client that he is about to feel a stick.	Client has better control over his anxiety when he knows what to expect.
14. Place thumb or forefinger of your nondominant hand 2.5 cm (1 inch) below site and pull client's skin taut toward you.	Stabilizes vein and prevents rolling during needle insertion.
15. Hold syringe or Vacutainer and needle at 15-30 degree angle from client's arm with bevel of needle up.	Reduces chance of penetrating both sides of vein during insertion. Bevel up causes less trauma to vein.
16. Slowly insert needle into vein.	Prevents puncture of entire vein.
17. With syringe, pull back gently on plunger while securing barrel. Hold Vacutainer securely and advance specimen tube into needle of holder.	Secure hold on syringe or Vacutainer prevents needle from advancing. Pulling on syringe plunger or inserting tube creates vacuum needed to draw blood into syringe or Vacutainer.

Steps	Rationale
18. Note flow of blood into syringe or tube.	If blood fails to appear, indicates that needle is not in vein or vacuum has been lost in specimen tube.
19. Obtain desired amount of blood.	Test results are more accurate when specified amount is drawn.
20. Once specimen obtained, release tourniquet.	Reduces bleeding at site when needle is withdrawn.
21. Remove needle from vein: Place gauze 2 × 2 or alcohol pad over venipuncture site without applying pressure. Using other hand, withdraw needle by pulling straight back from venipuncture site.	Pressure over needle can cause discomfort. Straight removal of needle from vein prevents injury to vein and other surrounding tissues.
22. Apply pressure to site.	Pressure controls bleeding. If client has been anticoagulated, pressure may be necessary for 3-5 minutes to prevent hematoma formation.
23. For blood obtained by syringe, transfer specimen to tube. Insert needle through stopper of blood tube and allow vacuum to fill tube. Do not force.	Vacuum present in specimen tube causes blood to enter. Forcing blood into tube can cause hemolysis.
24. For blood tubes containing additives, gently rotate back and forth 8-10 times.	Additives mixed to prevent clotting.
25. Inspect puncture site for bleeding and apply Band-Aid.	Keeps puncture site clean and controls final oozing.
26. Attach properly completed identification label to each tube, affix requisition, and send to lab.	Tests should be performed properly. Incorrect labeling can cause diagnostic error.

Steps	Rationale
27. Dispose of needles, syringes, soiled equipment and wash hands.	Reduces transmission of microorganisms.

Nurse Alert

Pressure must be applied to the venipuncture site in clients with a bleeding disorder or low platelet count or in those receiving anticoagulant therapy. It will decrease the risk of hematoma formation.

Client Teaching

If a woman has impaired lymphatic drainage (as may occur following a mastectomy), she should be instructed to tell care givers to avoid blood sampling from that arm. Impaired lymphatic drainage results in edema, and venipuncture in that extremity is difficult. Lack of lymphatic flow also predisposes the client to infection from skin puncture.

Pediatric Considerations

The nurse should not make numerous punctures in a child's arm for blood sampling. This can be extremely upsetting. A young child who requires venous sampling may need restraining by a staff member or parent. This will help immobilize the limb and prevent sudden movement that could result in serious injury to the blood vessel.

Geriatric Considerations

A frail elderly client's veins are fragile, and venipuncture becomes more difficult. The nurse should carefully assess such a client before venipuncture so he does not have to be repeatedly stuck with the needle. Because the elderly client's veins are fragile, bleeding may occur more easily in the tissues once the needle is withdrawn.

Venipuncture With an Angiocatheter For Initiating Intravenous Therapy

Venipuncture is a technique in which a vein is punctured transcutaneously by a sharp rigid stylet, such as an angiocatheter, or by a needle attached to a syringe. The major use of this technique is to initiate and maintain intravenous fluid therapy. In many settings the nurse has primary responsibility for initiating intravenous therapy with an angiocatheter.

Potential Nursing Diagnoses

Clients who require intravenous therapy with an angiocatheter may have one or more of the following nursing diagnoses:

Actual or potential fluid volume deficit related to prolonged vomiting, diarrhea, burns, or restricted intake

Potential alteration in cardiac output related to fluid volume excess

Anxiety related to impending needle stick

Alteration in comfort related to needle stick

Equipment

Correct solution

Infusion set

Intravenous tubing to deliver prescribed rate

Angiocatheter

Alcohol and povidone-iodine (Betadine) cleaning swabs

Tourniquet

Arm board
2 × 2 gauze and Betadine ointment
Tape that is cut and ready to use
Towel to place under client's hand
Intravenous pole
Razor (optional)

Steps	Rationale
1. Wash hands.	Reduces transmission of microorganisms.
2. Gather all equipment needed and bring it to bedside.	Maintains organization and avoids having to leave client to get more equipment. More than one of each piece of equipment is recommended in case a piece of sterile equipment becomes contaminated.
3. Organize equipment on clutter-free bedside stand or over-bed table.	Reduces risk of contamination and accidents.
4. Open sterile packages using aseptic technique.	Prevents contamination of sterile objects.
5. Check IV solution, using "five rights." Make sure that any prescribed additives (e.g., potassium or vitamins) have been added.	IV solutions are medications and should be double-checked at this point to reduce error.
▪ NOTE: When using bottled intravenous solution, remove metal cap and metal and rubber disks beneath cap.	Permits entry of infusion tubing into solution.
6. Have infusion set opened, maintaining sterility of both ends.	Prevents bacteria from entering infusion equipment and thus client's bloodstream.
7. Place roller clamp 2-4 cm (1-2 inches) below drip chamber.	Proximity of roller clamp to drip chamber allows more accurate regulation of flow rate.

Steps	Rationale
8. Move roller clamp up to *off* position. (Fig. 192)	Prevents accidental spillage of intravenous fluid on you, client, bed, or floor.
9. Insert infusion set into fluid bag:	
▪ Remove protective cover from intravenous bag without touching opening. (Fig. 193)	Maintains sterility of solution.
▪ Remove protector cap from insertion spike, not touching spike, and insert spike into opening of intravenous bag. (Fig. 194)	Prevents contamination of solution from contaminated insertion spike.
▪ Be sure that insertion spike is completely inserted into opening of intravenous bag. (Fig. 195)	Permits spike to puncture membrane at end of intravenous bag opening, thereby allowing fluid to flow from bag into tubing.
10. Fill infusion tubing:	
▪ Compress drip chamber and release.	Creates suction effect, and fluid enters drip chamber. Removes air from tubing and permits it to fill with solution.
▪ Remove needle protector and release roller clamp to allow fluid to travel from drip cham-	

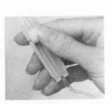

Fig. 192

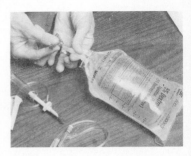

Fig. 193

Steps	Rationale
ber through needle adapter. Return roller clamp to *off* position. (Fig. 196)	
▪ Check tubing for air bubbles. If present, remove them by allowing more fluid to flow through tubing. Collect excess solution in basin and discard.	Large air bubbles can act as emboli.
▪ Replace needle protector.	Maintains sterility of system.

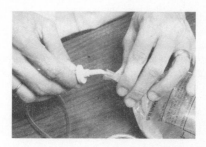

Fig. 194

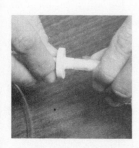

Fig. 195

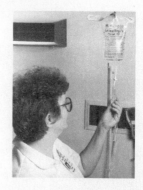

Fig. 196

Steps	Rationale
11. Select appropriate angio-catheter for venipuncture.	Size and type of needle depend on type of fluid to be infused and expected duration of therapy.
12. Select distal site in vein to be used.	If sclerosing or other damage to vein occurs, proximal site in same vein is still usable.
13. If large amount of body hair is present at insertion site, shave it off.	Reduces risk of contamination from bacteria that may be present on hair. Also makes removal of adhesive tape less painful.
14. If possible, place extremity in dependent position.	Permits dilation and visability of vein.
15. Place tourniquet 10-12 cm (5-6 inches) above insertion site. Tourniquet should obstruct venous, not arterial flow. (Fig. 197)	Diminished arterial flow prevents venous filling. Check for pressure of the distal pulse.
▪ NOTE: Do not tie tourniquet in a knot; use a loop tie.	Permits quick release of the tourniquet with one hand.

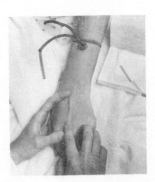

Fig. 197

Steps	Rationale
16. Select well-dilated vein. May help to have client make fist.	Muscle contraction increases venous distention.
■ NOTE: Be sure that needle adapter end of infusion set is nearby and on sterile gauze or towel.	Permits smooth quick connection of infusion tubing to the intravenous needle.
17. Clean insertion site with providone-iodine (Betadine) solution, followed by alcohol. Move in circular motion out from site 5 cm (2 inches). (Fig. 198)	Betadine is topical anti-infective; alcohol is topical antiseptic. Together these agents reduce skin surface bacteria.
18. Puncture vein using needle. Place needle at 30-degree angle with bevel up about 1 cm (½ inch) distal to actual site of venipuncture. Insert angiocatheter bevel-side up at 30-degree angle distal to actual site of venipuncture. (Figs. 199, 200)	Allows you to place needle parallel with vein. Thus, when vein is punctured, risk of complete penetration is reduced.

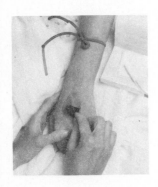

Fig. 198

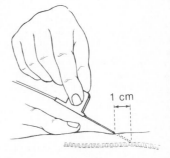

Fig. 199

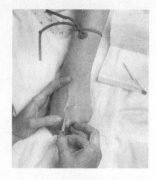

Fig. 200

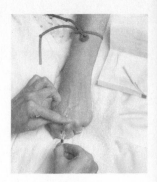

Fig. 201

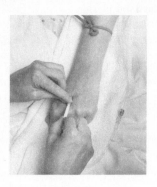

Fig. 202

Steps	Rationale
19. Look for blood return through angiocatheter, indicating that needle has entered vein. Remove needle from angiocatheter, leaving catheter in place. (Fig. 201)	Increased venous pressure from tourniquet increases backflow of blood into catheter or tubing. Small flexible catheter remains to permit entry of intravenous fluids.
20. Connect needle adapter of infusion set to hub of angiocatheter. To maintain sterility, do not touch entry point of needle adapter or hub of angiocatheter. (Fig. 202)	Prompt connection of infusion set maintains patency of vein.

Steps	Rationale
21. Stabilizing catheter with one hand, release tourniquet with other. (Fig. 203) Begin IV at ordered rate.	Permits venous flow. This prevents clotting in vein and obstruction of flow of solution.
22. Place Betadine ointment at point of catheter insertion. (Fig. 204)	Topical antiseptic-germicide reduces bacteria on skin. As a result risk of local or systemic infection is less.
23. Secure catheter	Prevents accidental removal from vein.
▪ Place narrow piece (½ inch) of tape under catheter. Cross tape over catheter. (Fig. 205)	
▪ Place second piece of narrow tape directly across catheter.	
▪ Place third piece of narrow tape under intravenous insertion needle adapter. Cross tape over infusion tubing. Place 2 × 2 gauze over catheter and secure it with 1-inch piece of tape.	Prevents accidental disconnection of infusion tubing.

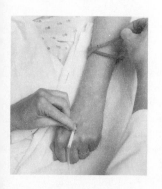

Fig. 203

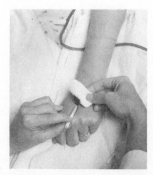

Fig. 204

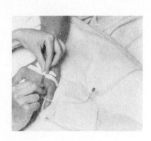

Fig. 205

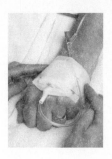

Fig. 206

Steps	Rationale
■ Secure infusion tubing to dressing with piece of 1-inch tape. (Fig. 206)	Further stabilizes connection of tubing to catheter.
24. Begin infusion.	Maintains patency of IV line.
25. Note date and time of placement of intravenous line. Dressing should be changed daily, following Steps 21 and 22.	Reduces bacteria in infusion tubing and on client's skin.
26. Record in nurse's notes type of fluid, insertion site, and type of catheter or needle used at time infusion began.	Documents that procedure was performed.

Nurse Alert

Venipuncture is contraindicated in a site that shows signs of infection, infiltration, or thrombosis. Infection is indicated by redness, tenderness, swelling, and warmth. Infiltration is identified by localized edema, blanching, and coolness of the surrounding tissues. Thrombosis is indicated by pain, swelling, and inflammation along the vein. To avoid displacement of the angiocatheter, an arm board is used.

Client Teaching

Clients and their families should be instructed not to move the extremity with the angiocatheter in place. Excessive motion can cause the angiocatheter to become displaced, resulting in an infiltration.

Pediatric Considerations

The nurse should not make numerous punctures in a child's arm for blood sampling. This can be extremely upsetting. A young child may need to be restrained to prevent infiltration and disruption of the intravenous flow rate.

Geriatric Considerations

The veins of elderly persons may be fragile, and consequently venipuncture is more difficult. In addition, frail elderly clients are at risk of infiltration and thrombosis due to irritation of the walls of the vein.

Regulating Intravenous Flow Rate

Once an intravenous infusion is in place and secured, the nurse has the responsibility of regulating its rate according to physician's orders. An infusion rate that is too slow can lead to further cardiovascular and circulatory collapse in a client who is dehydrated, in shock, or critically ill. A too rapid infusion rate can result in fluid overload. The nurse calculates the infusion rate to prevent incorrect fluid administration.

Potential Nursing Diagnoses

Clients in need of an intravenous infusion may have either of the following nursing diagnoses:

    Potential fluid volume deficit

    Potential fluid volume excess

Equipment

Paper and pencil

Watch with secondhand

Steps	Rationale
1. Read physician's orders and follow ''five rights'' to be sure that you have correct solution and proper additives.	IV fluids are medications; following the ''five rights'' decreases chance of medication error.
2. Intravenous fluids are usually ordered for 24-hour period, indicating how	Determines volume of fluid that should infuse hourly.

Steps	Rationale

long each liter of fluid
should run. For example
    Bottle 1—1000 ml
          D5W c̄ 20
          mEq KCl
          8 AM–4 PM
    Bottle 2—1000 ml
          D5W c̄ 20
          mEq KCl
          4 PM–12 MN
    Bottle 3—1000 ml
          D5W c̄ 20
          mEq KCl
          12 MN–8
          AM
    Total 24-hour IV in-
    take: 3000 ml

3. To determine hourly rate, divide volume by hours:

$$\frac{3000 \text{ ml}}{24} = 125 \text{ ml/hr}$$

Provides even infusion over 24 hours.

4. Intravenous fluid orders for 24-hour period may also be written as
    Bottle 1—1000 ml
          D5W c̄ 20
          mEq KCl
          8 AM–4 PM
    Bottle 2—1000 D5W
          c̄ 20 mEq
          KCl
          4 PM–12
          MN
    Bottle 3—500 D5W
          12 MN–8
          AM
Hourly rate would be

$$\frac{2000}{16} = 125 \text{ ml}$$ (8 AM–12 MN)

Fluid needs vary. Rate must be as ordered.

Steps	Rationale
$\dfrac{500}{8} = 63$ ml	(12 MN–8 AM)

5. Once hourly rate has been determined, minute rate is calculated based on drop factor of infusion set. Minidrip or microdrip infusion set has drop factor of 60 drops (gtt) per milliliter. Regular drip or macrodrip infusion set has drop factor of 15 gtt/ml

Allows you to calculate hourly flow rate based on this formula:

$$\dfrac{\text{Total volume} \times \text{Drop factor}}{\text{Infusion time in minutes}}$$

6. Using formula, calculate minute flow rates:

Bottle 1 (1000 ml c̄ 20 mEq KCl)

Microdrip

$$\dfrac{125 \text{ ml} \times 60 \text{ gtt/ml}}{60 \text{ minutes}}$$
$$= \dfrac{7500 \text{ gtt}}{60 \text{ min}}$$
$$= 125 \text{ gtt/min}$$

Volume is divided by time.

Macrodrip

$$\dfrac{125 \text{ ml} \times 15 \text{ gtt/ml}}{60 \text{ minutes}}$$
$$= 31\text{-}32 \text{ gtt/min}$$

7. Time the flow rate by counting drops in drip chamber for 1 minute by watch, then adjust roller clamp to increase or decrease speed of infusion. Check this rate hourly. (Figs. 207, 208)

Determines if fluids are being administered too slowly or too fast.

8. Place adhesive tape on intravenous bag next to volume markings. This figure is based on 125 ml in 8-hour period.

Time taping of intravenous bag gives you visual cue as to whether fluids are being administered at proper rate.

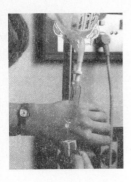

Fig. 207

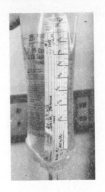

Fig. 208

Steps	Rationale
9. Record in nurse's notes if IV is patent and infusing on time.	Documents IV status and client's response.

Nurse Alert

An IV that fails to infuse on time may be an early sign of infiltration. If an infusion pump is used, the nurse should still monitor the rate of flow of the intravenous solution at least hourly. If intravenous fluids are excessively slow or fast, the physician should be contacted for revision of the intravenous flow rate before the flow is increased or decreased.

Client Teaching

The client should be instructed to report any tenderness or swelling at the venipuncture site.

Pediatric Considerations

Intravenous flows in children should always be maintained at the prescribed rate because fluid imbalances can occur rapidly. Pediatric settings usually require that infusion pumps or volume control devices be used with intravenous therapy.

Geriatric Considerations

Elderly clients with cardiovascular or renal disorders are at increased risk of fluid volume overload. The nurse must be extra careful to deliver an infusion at the prescribed rate of flow.

Changing Intravenous Solution

The nurse changes intravenous solutions using sterile technique to discontinue a specific solution or to remove an empty solution container and reconnect the tubing to a new container.

Potential Nursing Diagnoses

Clients requiring frequent changes in intravenous solutions may have either of the following nursing diagnoses:

Actual or potential fluid volume deficit

Actual or potential fluid volume excess

Equipment

Correct intravenous solution (or D5W to maintain patency of IV line)

Roller clamps

IV pole and bag

Steps	Rationale
1. Wash hands.	Reduces transmission of microorganisms.
2. Have next intravenous solution prepared at least 1 hour before it is needed. If solution is prepared in pharmacy, be sure that it has been delivered to floor. Check that it is correct and properly labeled.	Prevents finding empty intravenous bag without having replacement bag. Also prevents medication error.

Steps	Rationale
3. Prepare to change solution when it remains in neck of bag or bottle.	Prevents air from entering intravenous tubing and vein from clotting due to lack of intravenous flow.
4. Be sure that drip chamber is half full.	Provides intravenous fluid while bag is being changed.
5. Prepare new solution for hanging: ■ Plastic bag—Remove protective cover from entry site. ■ Glass bottle—Remove metal cap, metal disk, and rubber disk.	Permits quick, smooth, and organized change from old solution to new.
6. Move roller clamp to reduce flow rate.	Prevents solution remaining in drip chamber from emptying.
7. Remove old solution bag or bottle from intravenous pole.	Brings work to eye level.
8. Quickly remove spike from old container and, without touching tip, insert it in new container.	Reduces risk that solution in drip chamber (Step 3) will run dry. Also maintains sterility.
9. Hang new bag.	Allows gravity to assist with delivery of fluid.
10. Check for air in tubing.	Reduces risk of embolus.
11. Make sure that drip chamber contains solution.	Reduces risk that air will enter tubing.
12. Regulate flow rate as prescribed.	Maintains measures to restore fluid balance.
13. Record in nurse's notes amount and type of fluid infused and amount and type of new fluid.	Documents that solution has infused and new infusion has been started.

Nurse Alert

If the present intravenous solution is likely to run low before new IV orders are received, the nurse must either slow the present solution to 10 or 15 ml/hr to keep the vein open (KVO) or hang a small bag or bottle (250 ml) of D5W and run it at a KVO rate.

Client Teaching

Clients should be instructed to notify nursing personnel if they notice that their intravenous solution is running low.

Changing Infusion Tubing

An intravenous infusion tubing change is necessary daily to maintain sterility and patency of the IV line. It is especially important following a blood transfusion or infusion of a viscous solution.

Potential Nursing Diagnoses

Clients who require changing of infusion tubing may have one or more of the following nursing diagnoses:

    Actual or potential fluid volume excess
    Actual or potential fluid volume deficit
    Potential for injury related to infection

Equipment

New infusion tubing
New intravenous solution if tubing change is synchronized
    with initiation of new infusion

Steps	Rationale
1. Wash hands.	Reduces transmission of microorganisms.
2. Prepare new intravenous solution.	Easier and safer to change tubing at this time.
3. Open infusion set and move roller clamp to *off* position.	Prevents spillage of solution after bag or bottle is spiked
4. Place insertion spike in opening of new intravenous solution bag or bottle.	Permits flow from bag into tubing.
5. Hang bag on pole.	Frees both hands.
6. Compress and release drip chamber.	Allows drip chamber to fill with solution.
7. Open roller clamp, remove protective cap from needle adapter, and flush tubing with solution.	Removes air from tubing and replaces it with fluid.
8. Replace protective cap.	Maintains sterility of needle adapter.
9. Place new intravenous tubing, without protective cap, on sterile 2 × 2 gauze near client's intravenous site.	Provides smooth quick insertion of new tubing and solution.
10. Remove top of gauze dressing overlying IV site one piece at a time. Do not remove tape securing intravenous catheter or needle.	Reduces chance of accidental catheter or needle removal.
11. Turn roller clamp to *off* position on old tubing.	Prevents spillage of fluid as tubing is removed from needle hub.

Steps	Rationale
12. Stabilize hub of intravenous catheter or needle. Gently pull out old tubing. Maintaining stability of hub, insert needle adapter of new tubing into hub.	Prevents accidental displacement of catheter or needle.
13. Open roller clamp.	Permits new intravenous solution to enter catheter or needle.
14. Apply new dressing (see Skill 12-7).	Reduces risk of bacterial infection from skin.
15. Regulate intravenous drip according to physician's orders.	Maintains fluid and electrolyte balance.
16. Record in nurse's notes changing of tubing and solution.	Documents that measures to maintain sterility were carried out.
17. Wash your hands.	Reduces transmission of microorganisms.

Nurse Alert

An intravenous tubing change is easier if the nurse organizes it to occur when a new solution bag is being hung. There are times, however, when it is not possible to have the two procedures occur simultaneously, as when tubing is accidentally punctured with a needle.

Changing an Intravenous Infusion Dressing

The dressing over an intravenous insertion site is changed daily so it can be inspected for possible infection or early infiltration. In addition, daily dressing changes reduce the chance of infection at the site.

Potential Nursing Diagnoses

Clients who require intravenous dressing changes may have either or both of the following nursing diagnosis:

Potential for injury related to infection

Impairment of skin integrity related to venipuncture site

Equipment

Tape—cut and ready to use

Alcohol and povidone-iodine (Betadine) cleaning swabs

2 × 2 gauze pads

4 × 4 gauze sponges (optional)

Betadine ointment

Self-adhesive elastic film (Op-Site, Tegaderm)

Steps	Rationale

Gauze Dressing

1. Wash hands.

Reduces transmission of microorganisms.

2. Remove old tape and gauze one piece at a time, leaving tape that secures intravenous needle or catheter in place.

Prevents accidental displacement of catheter or needle.

3. Gently remove tape securing needle or catheter. Stabilize needle or catheter with one hand.

Exposes venipuncture site. Stabilization prevents accidental displacement of catheter or needle.

4. Clean insertion site with povidone-iodine (Betadine) solution followed by alcohol.

Betadine is a topical anti-infective; alcohol is a topical antiseptic. Together these agents reduce skin surface bacteria.

5. Clean in circular motion, gradually moving away from venipuncture site.

Prevents cross-contamination from skin bacteria near venipuncture site.

6. Place Betadine ointment on venipuncture site.

Reduces bacteria on skin and therefore risk of local or systemic infection.

7. Secure intravenous catheter and dressing (Skill 12-3).

Prevents accidental removal of catheter from vein and stabilizes connection of infusion to catheter.

8. Write date and time of dressing change on dressing itself.

Provides visual documentation of exactly when dressing was changed.

Transparent Dressing

1. Wash hands.

Reduces transmission of microorganisms.

2. Remove dressing, applying support to underlying angiocatheter or butterfly needle.

Prevents accidental displacement of catheter or needle.

Steps	Rationale
3. Observe insertion site for redness tenderness, edema.	Indicates possible inflammation or infiltration.
4. Clean insertion site with povidone-iodine (Betadine) solution followed by alcohol.	Betadine is a topical anti-infective; alcohol a topical antiseptic. Together these agents reduce skin surface bacteria.

5. Apply new transparent dressing:
  ■ Remove protective covering on dressing.
  ■ Grasp dressing by corners.
  ■ Apply in direction of hair growth.
	Serves as barrier to external fluids and bacteria. Also allows underlying skin to "breathe." Dressing requires changing everyday.

6. Record in nurse's notes day and time of change.	Documents when dressing change occurred.

Nurse Alert

As is true of any sterile dressing, when an intravenous dressing becomes moist, it is contaminated and must be changed.

Geriatric Considerations

Because of the increased fragility of the skin in older adults, the nurse must predetermine if hypoallergenic paper tape should be used to secure the IV dressing. In the presence of sensitive skin, she should be careful to use only enough tape to secure the dressing.

Administering a Blood Transfusion

Blood products are ordered by the physician to restore circulatory blood volume, improve hemoglobin, or correct serum protein levels. The administration of blood or blood components is a nursing procedure.

Potential Nursing Diagnoses

Clients who require blood transfusions may have either or both of the following nursing diagnoses:

Actual or potential fluid volume deficit related to loss of blood volume

Altered cardiac output related to decreased circulatory blood volume

Equipment

In addition to that used to initiate an IV infusion

Normal saline IV solution, 0.9%

Infusion set with inline filter

Large catheter (18 or 19 gauge)

Correct blood product

Another nurse to double-check correct blood product with correct client

Steps	Rationale
1. Wash hands.	Reduces transmission of microorganisms.
2. Explain procedure to client. Determine if there has been any prior transfusion and note reactions, if any.	Clients who have had blood transfusion in past may have greater fear of transfusion.
3. Ask client to immediately report any of following symptoms: chills, headache, itching, rash.	These can be signs of a transfusion reaction. Prompt reporting and discontinuation of transfusion will help minimize reaction.
4. Be sure that client has signed any necessary consent forms.	Some agencies require clients to sign consent forms before receiving any blood component transfusions.
5. Establish intravenous line with large (18 or 19 gauge) catheter.	Permits infusion of whole blood and prevents hemolysis.
6. Use infusion tubing that has in-line filter. Tubing should also be Y-type administration set. (Fig. 209)	Filter removes any debris and tiny clots from blood. Using Y-type set permits (a) administration of additional products or volume expanders easily and (b) immediate infusion of 0.9% sodium chloride solution after completion of initial infusion.

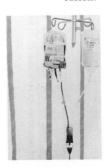

Fig. 209

Steps	Rationale
7. Hang solution container of 0.9% normal saline to be administered after blood infusion.	Prevents hemolysis of red blood cells.
8. Follow agency protocol in obtaining blood products from blood bank. Request blood when you are ready to use it.	Whole blood or packed red blood cells must remain in a cold (1°-6° C) environment.
9. With another nurse, correctly identify blood product and client:	One nurse reads out loud while other nurse listens and double-checks information.
▪ Check compatibility tag attached to blood bag and information on bag itself.	Verifies that ABO group, Rh type, and unit number match.
▪ For whole blood, check ABO group and Rh type (on client's chart).	Verifies that they match those on compatibility tag and blood bag.
▪ Double-check blood product with physician's order.	Verifies correct blood component.
▪ Check expiration date on bag.	After 21 days, blood has only 70% to 80% of its original cells and 23 mEq/L of potassium.*
▪ Inspect blood for clots.	Anticoagulant, citrate-phosphate-dextrose (CPD), is added to blood and permits preserved blood to be stored for 21 days. Newer anticoagulant, citrate-phosphate-dextrose-adenine (CPD-A), allows storage for 35 days.* If clots are present, return blood to blood bank.

*Data from Metheny, N.M., and Snively, W.D., Jr.: Nurse's handbook of fluid balance, ed. 4, Philadelphia, 1983, J.B. Lippincott Co.

Steps	Rationale
▪ Ask client's name. Check armband.	Verifies correct client. Do not administer blood to client without an arm band. Identification name and number on wristband must be identical to those on blood compatibility tag.
10. Monitor client's vital signs:	
▪ Take baseline recording before administering transfusion.	Verifies client's pretransfusion temperature, pulse, blood pressure, and respirations.
▪ Check every 5 minutes for first 15 minutes of transfusion.	Documents any change in vital sign status, which could indicate early warning of transfusion reaction.
▪ Observe client for flushing, itching, dyspnea, hives, or rash.	This may indicate an early sign of a transfusion reaction.
11. Begin transfusion:	
▪ Prime infusion line with 0.9% normal saline.	Prevents hemolysis.
▪ Begin transfusion slowly by first filling in-line filter.	If filter is not filled, transfusion will not flow properly.
▪ Adjust rate to 2 ml/min for first 15 minutes. Remain with client. If you suspect a reaction, *stop* transfusion and notify blood bank and physician.	
12. Maintain prescribed infusion rate, using infusion pumps if necessary.	Pumps maintain the prescribed rate.
13. Continually observe for adverse reactions.	Can occur at any point during transfusion.
14. Record in nurse's notes administration of blood or blood product.	Documents that procedure was performed.

Nurse Alert

Complaints of itching, flushing, dyspnea, hives, or rash or changes in vital signs could signify a transfusion reaction. Immediately stop the transfusion, notify the physician, and maintain patency of the IV catheter with 0.9% normal saline at a KVO (keep vein open) rate.

Client Teaching

Instruct the client to notify nursing personnel if he feels uncomfortable at any time during or immediately after the transfusion. Reactions can occur immediately or up to 6 hours after the transfusion.

Pediatric Considerations

Transfusions in the infant and child are given at a slower rate. In the infant exchange transfusions are done by a physician, withdrawing and infusing the same volume with each procedure. In the child 50 ml of blood is given over 30 minutes. If no reaction occurs, the flow rate is increased to allow the remainder of the blood to infuse over 2 hours.

Geriatric Considerations

The older client may be at risk of circulatory overload because of preexisting cardiopulmonary disease, which tends to be more common in the geriatric population.

Changing a Total Parenteral Nutrition Dressing

Dressings for total parenteral nutrition (TPN) sites should be changed at least every 48 hours. Some institutions may state that dressings over central veins such as the subclavian should be changed every 24 hours while peripheral sites can be changed every 48 hours. The TPN dressing change is similar to the IV infusion dressing change (Skill 12-7) except that the nurse should wear a mask and gloves.

Potential Nursing Diagnoses

Clients requiring change of a total parenteral nutrition dressing may have either or both of the following nursing diagnoses:

Alteration in nutrition: less than body requirements
Potential for injury related to infection at infusion site

Equipment

Sterile gloves
Sterile barrier
Sterile Betadine (povidone-iodine) swabs
Mask
Sterile alcohol swabs
Betadine ointment
2 × 2 gauze pads
4 × 4 gauze pads
Tape
Sterile cotton-tipped catheter

Steps	Rationale
1. Collect equipment.	Prevents your needing to leave bedside to collect more supplies.
2. Wash hands.	Reduces transmission of microorganisms.
3. Apply mask.	Prevents transmission of airborne bacteria to insertion site.
4. Remove old dressing slowly, one layer at a time. Touch only outside or corners of dressing.	Careful removal prevents accidental dislodging of catheter and contamination of puncture site.
5. Assess venipuncture site for infection and catheter for knots or kinks.	Prevents systemic contamination that would occur by administering fluid through contaminated site. Also maintains catheter patency.
6. Spread sterile barrier and place supplies, using sterile technique, on field. Don sterile gloves (Skill 5-6).	Maintains sterility of field.
7. Clean the area with alcohol swabs beginning at catheter site and moving outward in circular motion at least 5 cm (2 inches). Repeat two more times. Follow this procedure using povidone-iodine (Betadine) swabs.	Removes bacteria from venipuncture site. Circular motion outward prevents cross-contamination with other skin bacteria.
8. Using sterile cotton-tipped applicator, apply Betadine ointment directly over catheter exit site.	Reduces risk of bacterial infection.
9. Cover site with 2 × 2 and 4 × 4 gauze pads, and cover these completely with tape.	Airtight dressing reduces entry of airborne bacteria.

Steps	Rationale
10. Date and initial dressing.	Identifies to nursing and medical personnel when dressing change occurred.
11. Dispose of mask and soiled equipment.	
12. Wash your hands.	Reduces transmission of microorganisms.
13. Record in client's chart dressing change.	Provides documentation of procedure.

Nurse Alert

Total parenteral nutrition solutions are high in glucose, and as a result they are irritants to the veins. Peripheral veins, which are commonly used for the infusion of lipids and dilute glucose-protein hydrolysates, are at great risk of inflammation and irritation. Therefore the nurse should continually assess these sites for irritation. Due to the high concentration of glucose in TPN solutions, it may be necessary to monitor the client's blood glucose levels regularly as well.

Pediatric Considerations

Most pediatric institutions require that the infusion tubing and dressing be changed under meticulous aseptic technique every 24 hours.

APPENDIX

Approved Nursing Diagnoses

- Activity intolerance
- Activity intolerance, potential
- Airway clearance, ineffective
- Anxiety
- Bowel elimination, alteration in: constipation
- Bowel elimination, alteration in: diarrhea
- Bowel elimination, alteration in: incontinence
- Breathing pattern, ineffective
- Cardiac output, alteration in: decreased
- Comfort, alteration in: pain
- Communication, impaired: verbal
- Coping, family: potential for growth
- Coping, ineffective family: compromised
- Coping, ineffective family: disabling
- Coping, ineffective individual
- Diversional activity, deficit
- Family process, alteration in (formerly Family dynamics)
- Fear
- Fluid, volume, alterations in: excess
- Fluid volume deficit, actual
- Fluid volume deficit, potential
- Gas exchange, impaired
- Grieving, anticipatory
- Grieving, dysfunctional

From Kim, M.J., et al., editors: Classification of nursing diagnoses: proceedings of the fifth National Conference, St. Louis, 1984, The C.V. Mosby Co.

- Health maintenance, alteration in
- Home maintenance management, impaired
- Injury, potential for: (poisoning, potential for; suffocation, potential for; trauma, potential for)
- Knowledge deficit (specify)
- Mobility, impaired physical
- Noncompliance (specify)
- Nutrition, alteration in: less than body requirements
- Nutrition, alteration in: more than body requirements
- Nutrition, alteration in: potential for more than body requirements
- Oral mucous membrane, alteration in
- Parenting, alteration in: actual
- Parenting, alteration in: potential
- Powerlessness
- Rape trauma syndrome
- Self-care deficit: feeding, bathing/hygiene, dressing/grooming, toileting
- Self-concept, disturbance in: body image, self-esteem, role performance, personal identity
- Sensory-perceptual alteration: visual, auditory, kinesthetic, gustatory, tactile, olfactory
- Sexual dysfunction
- Skin integrity, impairment of: actual
- Skin integrity, impairment of: potential
- Sleep pattern disturbance
- Social isolation
- Spiritual distress (distress of the human spirit)
- Thought processes, alteration in
- Tissue perfusion, alteration in: cerebral, cardiopulmonary, renal, gastrointestinal, peripheral
- Urinary elimination, alteration in patterns
- Violence, potential for: self-directed or directed at others

BIBLIOGRAPHY

Aman, R.A.: Treating the patient, not the constipation, Am. J. Nurs. **80:**1634, 1980.

American Heart Association: Recommendations for human blood pressure determination by sphygmomanometers, Dallas, 1980, The Association.

Anders, J.E.: Topicals: a welter of options calls for refined application techniques, RN **45:**32, 1982.

Bates, P.: A troubleshooter's guide to indwelling catheters, RN **44:**63, 1981.

Bennett, J.V.: Incidence and nature of endemic and epidemic nosocomial infections. In Bennett, J.F., and Brachman, P.S., editors: Hospital infection, Boston, 1979, Little, Brown & Co.

Bielski, M.: Preventing infection in the catheterized patient. Nurs. Clin. North Am. **15:**703, 1980.

Bilger, A.J., and Greene, E.H.: Winger's protective body mechanics: a manual for nurses, New York, 1973, Springer Publishing Co., Inc.

Blainey, C.G.: Site selection in taking body temperatures, Am. J. Nurs. **74:**1859, 1974.

Blodgett, D.: Manual of respiratory care procedures, Philadelphia, 1980, J.B. Lippincott Co.

Bradley, J., and Edenberg, M.A.: Communication in the nursing context, East Norwalk, Conn., 1982, Appleton-Century-Crofts.

Bruno, P.: The nature of wound healing: implications for nursing practice, Nurs. Clin. North Am. **14:**667, 1979.

Carden, R.G.: The ins and outs of contact lenses, RN **48:**48, Feb. 1985.

Clark, J.B., et al: Pharmacological basis of nursing practice, ed. 2, St. Louis, 1986, The C.V. Mosby Co.

Contact lens removal, JEN **6:**15, 1980.

Corbett, J.V.: Laboratory tests in nursing practice, East Norwalk, Conn., 1982, Appleton-Century-Crofts.

Cuzzell, J.Z.: Wound care forum: Artful solutions to chronic problems, Am. J. Nurs. 85:162, Feb. 1985.

Davis, M.: Getting to the root of the problem: hair grooming techniques for black patients, Nursing 77 7:60, 1977.

Davis, N.M., and Cohen, M.R.: Learning from mistakes: 20 tips for avoiding medication errors, Nursing 82 12:65, 1982.

Ebersole, P., and Hess, P.: Toward healthy aging: human needs and nursing response, ed. 2, St. Louis, 1984, The C.V. Mosby Co.

Egan, G.: The skilled helper, Monterey, Calif., 1975, Brookes/Cole Publishing Co.

Ek, A., and Boman, G.: A descriptive study of pressure sores: the prevalence of pressure sores and the characteristics of patients, J. Adv. Nurs. 7:51, 1982.

Enelow, A., and Scott, S.: Interviewing and patient care, ed. 2, New York, 1979, Oxford University Press, Inc.

Eoff, M.J., and Joyce, B.: Temperature measurements in children, Am. J. Nurs. 81:1010, 1981.

Erickson, R.: Oral temperature differences in relation to thermometer and technique, Nurs. Res. 29:157, 1980.

Felton, C.L.: Hypoxemia and oral temperatures, Am. J. Nurs. 78:57, 1978.

Flynn, M.E., and Rover, D.T.: Wound healing mechanisms, Am. J. Nurs. 82:1544, 1982.

Francis, B.: Hot and cold therapy, J. Nurs. Care 15:18, 1982.

Gannon, E.P., and Kadezabek, E.: Giving your patients meticulous mouth care, Nursing 80 10:14, 1980.

Garner, J.S., and Simmons, B.P.: CDC guidelines for isolation precautions in hospitals, Infect. Control 4(4):249, 1983.

Gordon, M: Nursing diagnosis: process and application, New York, 1982, McGraw-Hill Book Co.

Graves, R.D., and Markarian, M.F.: Three minute time interval when using an oral mercury-in-glass thermometer with or without J temp sheaths, Nurs. Res. 29:232, 1980.

Hanawalt, A., and Troutman, K.: If your patient has a hearing aid, Am. J. Nurs. 84:900, 1984.

Hargins, C.O., and Larson, E.: Infection control guidelines for prevention of hospital acquired infections, Am. J. Nurs. 81:2175, 1981.

Holder, L.: Hearing aids, handle with care, Nursing 82 12:64, April, 1982.

Hudson, M.P.: Safeguard your elderly patient's health through accurate physical assessment, Nursing 83 13:58, 1983.

Iveson-Iveson, J.: The art of communication, Nurs. Mirror, p. 47, Feb. 2, 1984.

Jones, S.: Simpler and safer tube-feeding techniques, RN **47**:40, Oct. 1984.

Kerr, J.C., et al.: Pressure sores: distinguishing fact from fiction, Can. Nurse **77**:23, July-Aug. 1981.

Kim, M.J., et al., editors: Classification of nursing diagnoses: proceedings of the fifth National Conference, St. Louis, 1984, The C.V. Mosby Co.

Kim, M.J., et al.: Pocket guide to nursing diagnoses, St. Louis, 1984, The C.V. Mosby Co.

Kirillof, L.H., and Tibbals, S.C.: Drugs for asthma, a complete guide, Am. J. Nurs. **83**:55, 1983.

Kosiak, M.: Etiology of decubitus ulcers, Arch. Phys. Med. Rehab. **42**:19, 1961.

LaVelle, B.E., and Snyder, M.: Differential conduction of cold through barriers: Ace bandages, padded Ace bandages, and compression dressings in the management of acute soft tissue trauma, J Adv. Nurs. **10**(1):55, 1985.

Levin, P.: Safeguarding your patients against periodontal disease, RN **36**:38, 1973.

Little, D.E., and Carnevali, D.C.: Nursing care planning, ed. 3, Philadelphia, 1983, J.B. Lippincott Co.

Longworth, J.C.D.: Psychophysiological effects of slow stroke back massage in normotensive females, ANS **4**:44, July 1982.

Luce, J.M., et al.: Intensive respiratory care, Philadelphia, 1984, W.B. Saunders Co.

McConnell, E.A.: The subtle art of really good injections, RN **45**:24, 1982.

Michelson, D.: How to give a good back rub, Am. J. Nurs. **78**:1197, 1978.

Millam, D.A.: How to get into hard-to-stick veins, RN **48**:34, Apr. 1985.

Morley, M.: 16 steps to better decubitus ulcer care, Can. Nurse **77**:29, July-Aug. 1981.

Nichols, G.A., and Kucha, D.H.: Taking adult temperature: oral measurement, Am. J. Nurs. **72**:1090, 1972.

Olson, E.V.: The hazards of immobility, Am. J. Nurs. **67**:779, 1967.

Pollack, S.: Wound healing: a review. II. Environmental factors affecting wound healing, J. Enterostom. Ther. **9**:14, 1982.

Ramos, L.Y.: Oral hygiene for the elderly, Am. J. Nurs. **81**:1468, 1981.

Raudseff, E.: Seven ways to cure communication breakdowns, Nurs. Life, p. 51, Jan.-Feb. 1984.

Retting, F.M., and Southby, J.R.: Using different body positions to reduce discomfort from dorsogluteal injection, Nurs. Res. **31**:219, 1982.

Saxton, D.F., et al.: Addison Wesley manual of nursing practice, Los Altos, Calif., 1983, Addison Wesley Co.

Shapiro, B.A., et al.: Clinical application of blood gases, ed. 2, Chicago, 1977, Year Book Medical Publishers, Inc.

Simmons, B.P.: CDC guidelines for prevention of surgical wound infections, Am. J. Infect. Control **11**:133, 1983.

Surr, C.W.: New blood glucose products. I, Nursing 83 **13**:42, 1983.

Surr, C.W.: New blood glucose monitoring products. II, Nursing 83 **13**:58, 1983.

Tanner, S.: IV bolus leaves no room for error, RN **44**:54, 1981.

Thomas, D.O.: Fever in children, RN **48**:18, Dec. 1985.

Thompson, D.R.: Recording patients' blood pressure: a review, J. Adv. Nurs. **6**:283, 1981.

Whaley, L.F., and Wong, D.L.: Nursing care of infants and children, ed. 2, St. Louis, 1983, The C.V. Mosby Co.

Williams, W.W.: CDC guidelines for infection control in hospital personnel, Infect. Control **4**(4):325, 1983.

Williamson, M.L.: Reducing post-catheterization bladder dysfunction in reconditioning, Nurs. Res. **31**:28, 1982.